Rev It Up!

The Lifestyle Diet that Puts YOU in the Driver's Seat

Tammy Beasley, RD, CSSD, LD

Rev It Up!

The Lifestyle Diet that Puts YOU in the Driver's Seat

Written by Tammy Beasley, RD, CSSD, LD
Registered, licensed dietitian, certified specialist in sports dietetics, certified Spinning instructor

Cover design by Emily Martinez, www.thebigpix.com

Distributed by Rev It Up Fitness, LLC. Printed by American Printing Company, Birmingham, Alabama,USA.

ISBN 978-0-615-33769-2

This publication is designed to provide information in regard to the subject matter covered. It is distributed with the understanding that the writer, editor, and publisher are not engaged in offering medical advice. Medical Warning: This manual proposes a program of physical and dietary recommendations for the reader to follow. However, before starting this or any other wellness program, you should consult your physician.

Visit us on the Web: www.revitupfitness.com

Rev It Up! is dedicated to all the clients with whom I have worked over the last 25 years. Thank you for sharing your lives with me. Each of you has contributed to this manuscript, and I am grateful and blessed to have had the privilege to work with you.

To my parents, thank you for setting the example of following your heart and never giving up. And to my husband, Dan, and sons, Adam and Luke–you have never failed to support my dream to one day, indeed, put in print the message of "Rev It Up!" that I have learned to live and share over the years. It's been an eight year journey to see this through, and thank you for walking it with me!

Contents

What the Experts are Saying

"Tammy Beasley is eminently qualified to help improve the overall health and well-being of individuals with a wide range of nutrition–related issues. Her rigorous and comprehensive technical education and clinical training in the field of dietetics, as well as her unique professional and personal experiences, have positioned her as a leading authority in the art and science of 'eating and living well'."
Dean June Henton, College of Human Sciences
Auburn University

"Just the guidance you need to put into action strategies for life! Tammy Beasley, Licensed Registered Dietitian, has easily translated evidence-based science for you into a meaningful, realistic roadmap for a life-long journey of healthy living. Tammy lives the life that she is sharing in this book–and serves as a living example both professionally and healthfully as true testament that the route you take next will be forever life-changing. Now....full speed ahead!'
Susan C. Scott, RD, LD
President and CEO, SCS Nutrition Consulting
2008 Outstanding Dietitian, Alabama Dietetic Association

"I love Rev It Up! and have found in it the one source for most all the information I need to help my patients get beyond 'I'm on a diet' thinking to 'I can live a healthy lifestyle' thinking. Rev It Up! has solid nutritional information presented in a creative, incremental, organized and timely way. It is comprehensive, yet easily understandable for my patients. The program has a built-in schedule and logbook to assist my clients in tracking their progress through the program. After working through the program, my clients are well-equipped to become independent 'non dieters' who are able to make healthy lifestyle decisions for themselves. I like the analogy drawn between a car engine and our 'metabolic machines' and predict Rev It Up! will become a household word across the country. I think of it as my personal wellness assistant."
Ginger Ryan Combs, RD, LD
Clinical Dietitian

"Rev It Up! is not a fad diet; it's an eating strategy and fitness prescription for healthy living that is essential for regaining control of your life. This book is a must have if you are serious about changing your eating habits, losing weight and getting fit."
> Officer Chris Hluzek
> Police Academy and S.W.A.T. Fitness Instructor

"I started teaching Rev It Up! in January 2007 as part of my employee wellness program. Interesting note from a participant after the first week as he said, 'You haven't told me what to eat yet. That's different and I LIKE IT!' Rev It Up! is about overall real-life changes and not following a strict diet. It's a very positive program."
> Janelle Campbell, MS, RD, CDE
> Clinical Dietitian

"Tammy's expertise in re-teaching clients to trust their bodies, understand hunger and fullness, and accept and appreciate their bodies' needs has been invaluable to my clients. Her personal warmth and caring commitment to clients as well as her approach to wellness have been an integral part of my clients' ability to succeed."
> Dana Summers, LPC, NBCC
> Licensed Professional Counselor

"Tammy Beasley is an excellent clinical nutritionist. I am impressed with her knowledge and great communication skills. She has created a fantastic tool in the Rev It Up! program for achieving a safe and effective approach to weight loss."
> Raetta Bevan Fountain, MD
> Gastroenterologist

"As a physical therapist, I was excited to find such a dynamic and comprehensive health and wellness program. Having been through several nationally recognized weight-loss programs in the past, I feel this program is far superior in helping the client truly make a lifestyle change. This catch phrase is often alluded to in other programs, but Rev It Up! addresses all aspects of a healthy lifestyle including nutrition, fitness, and tackling the tough psychosocial components. Education is a cornerstone of the program, providing

sound, in-depth nutrition and fitness information in an easy-to-understand, easy-to-follow format which allows the client to make smart health decisions in real-life situations. The program is safe, effective, and more importantly, empowering."
  Janine Nesin, PT, DPT
  Physical Therapist

What Rev It Up! Alumni are Saying

"I have dieted my entire adult life–literally moving from one to the next searching for the 'one' that works. I heard about Rev It Up! and thought, 'Maybe this one will work?' My goal was no longer just weight loss. I wanted to eat like normal people. I can't express in words the difference this program has made in my life. No longer is a food or food group off limits. I eat-REAL food! I have gained so much confidence in myself and my choices. People see change in me, not just in size, but in my smile, too."
     Rebecca

"This program is a real eye opener. Can't believe what I did not know! We (my wife and I) can't stop talking about it. Probably the most dynamic program I've ever experienced. Rev It Up! makes sense, and really works...(written in 2002) (and again in 2007)...*"Many if not all of the Rev It Up! principles have been incorporated in our everyday living experiences and our lives. I cannot believe I 'did not know' how much I did not know about nutrition, exercise, and the value of how you eat and what you eat. Barbara and I have lost approximately 15 and 24 pounds, respectively, from the beginning of the program and we have managed to maintain 100% of that loss (five years later!). The program had a tremendous positive influence on our lives in terms of overall health and wellness. We learned the positive benefits of exercise and more specifically eating right, i.e. fuel for the body (I will never forget that session!)."*
     Al and Barbara

"Thank you for introducing me to my new life! Until now, I didn't know what it was like to have any self-confidence or look in the mirror and be able to think...'you look pretty good today!'"
     M.H.

"In our search for a diet and exercise program, my wife and I were interested in something different. We wanted something that stressed the science of diet and weight loss more than scales and calorie counting. We wanted to know how best to integrate exercise with correct eating habits. We wanted a program that was interesting and

worthwhile. We found Rev It Up! to fill these needs and more, and we recommend it as an excellent foundation for healthy living."
       Dr. R.W.

"I do not consider myself on a diet or doing without any foods I want at times. Rev It Up! is a way of life for me. I am mentally feeling in control again and physically am without the health problems that the 60's usually bring – no heart problems, no diabetes, and no cholesterol problems."
       Joyce

"Rev It Up! has taught me that there is a smart way to eat those foods I love and not feel guilty. It's also taught me to exercise smarter, too!"
       Mary

"Because of what I learned from Rev It Up!, I was able to apply the principles even while I was pregnant. I ate healthy (with the exception of just a few cravings!) and only gained 25 pounds during my entire pregnancy."
       Nikki

"I can't tell you how much I am enjoying Rev It Up! It seems to be giving me the freedom to eat healthy, eat when I'm hungry, eat without remorse, eat until I'm full. It has quieted the sugar cravings and stopped the binges in the evening. If just those two things can be conquered for the long haul, it is a miracle! No one has put it in a comprehensive, step-by-step format for me before. I can understand it, follow it, and there's really no desire to deviate–something I always felt the urge to do with other plans."
       Rose

"Rev It Up! is a more realistic and natural approach to changing my eating habits instead of a 'rigid denial' or chemical driven method like so many others. I also like the concept of the challenges, allowing me to focus on one aspect of change at a time."
       Julie

"Rev It Up! is the best money I have ever spent. I tell everyone about the program. The best benefit I received was freedom from cravings. I lost 10 pounds while working the program and have maintained 34 pounds of weight loss since then!"
Cheryl

"With all the gimmick and fad diets out there, this is actually a wellness program that doesn't make me feel deprived or that I'm on a diet."
J.D.

A Note from the Author

Rev It Up! was created after years of counseling hundreds of clients on two different ends of the wellness spectrum and hearing myself sharing the same information with all of them. These clients ranged from those with eating disorder struggles on one end to the elite athletes on the other end, and the chronic dieters and recreational athletes who were in the middle somewhere. The clients struggling with disordered eating needed to look inside out–to understand how and why their bodies were responding to their eating and exercise obsessions-and learn how to communicate with their bodies again through hunger, fullness, and embracing the goal of wellness vs. a specific body weight. The chronic dieter and recreational athlete-male, female, young and old–were in the middle of the spectrum with their own struggles about weight and fitness. And on the opposite end, the dedicated, competitive athletes came wanting to know as many hard facts, figures, and specific meal plans as possible to meet their fitness demands.

The great majority of consumer information available to the two opposite ends of the spectrum does not often overlap. Yet I found that the competitive athlete benefited from looking beyond meal plans to the "why" and "how" of metabolism-and slowing down to explore hunger/fullness cues completed the wellness picture. At the same time, I found that the eating disorder client benefited from knowing some simple, practical but specific guidelines on when and what to eat to help reduce the fear of food while exploring the emotions behind specific choices. And the chronic dieter and recreational athletes also gained new confidence learning and practicing these same principles-and broadened their perspective of wellness in general, their own bodies in detail.

Thus, Rev It Up! was born as a program for women and men that approached wellness by looking at metabolism first – HOW the body works-and WHY the traditional way of "doing diets" isn't enough. Is the educational component of the program new in the truths that are presented? Not really-to live well, an individual must fuel and move the body appropriately. But is it new in its approach? YES! The body as a car, metabolism as the engine, and food and fluid as the fuel–

with all the specific nuances of car maintenance and parts, from the fuel gauge, rear-view mirror, battery charge, oil change, and more. The car analogy runs throughout the entire program, which is progressive from week to week, building on the principles learned in a step-by-step approach. It's user-friendly, simple in presentation but complex in its power to change a person's perspective of living well!

I invite you to experience Rev It Up! for yourself. Join the hundreds before you who have made a difference in their own life by learning and living the Rev It Up! principles. I look forward to partnering with you to make a difference in your health, and welcome any opportunity to hear from you as you work the principles, see the changes, and feel the difference.

In health,

Tammy

Rev It Up!

The Lifestyle Diet that Puts YOU in the Driver's Seat

Introduction

Welcome to Rev It Up! Congratulations on investing in your future by learning how to lead a new lifestyle-not just follow a diet plan. You may be wondering how this program is different from any others. Can it make a lasting difference? Can you really learn to LIVE a new healthy lifestyle, or will this be another temporary change that won't last?

If you have ever felt that you and your body are moving in opposite directions from each other, this is the program for you! Rev It Up! is designed to help you take an inside look at your relationship with your own body and learn how to get on the same track again. Learn how to communicate with each other again. You may be surprised to discover how many ways your body "talks" and responds to your messages every day.

How do you get on the same track again with your body? Your health? Let's begin by thinking about your favorite car. What model is it? Do you have a specific color in mind for the exterior? The interior? Pretend you have been given this specific car, and it is yours to care for and maintain. You can make changes to the exterior, and the outside of your car will look better for awhile. But "outside" changes only cover up and disguise any real problems inside the engine. A new set of tires or a brand new coat of paint can dress things up but a neglected engine will stop your car in its tracks every time. You don't have to read the driver's manual or follow the maintenance guidelines, but if you want your "dream car" to perform as long as possible, you will.

You probably know where this is going now, don't you? Of course you might not agree that your body is the "dream car" you have always wanted, at least not now, but it is a special car, the only one of its kind. Designed specifically for you. And it is yours to keep, care for, and maintain.

So here's the analogy: Your body is the car, your metabolism is its engine, and food is its fuel. Consider this program your driver's manual, full of instructions, suggested tools to use, and reminders to guide you along the road. You CAN understand what your body's signals mean and how to respond. You can KNOW the signs of wear and tear, when to slow down or speed up, and when a tune-up is necessary. And you can keep your body in good, even excellent, condition to keep performing at its best.

Program Principles:
How to Use This Driver's Manual!

Rev It Up! is an eight week wellness program designed to help you develop a healthy partnership with your body. It incorporates eating and exercise strategies to achieve a more balanced healthy lifestyle and a more efficient metabolism rate. Sounds great, right? But before you can learn how to make simple changes to improve your metabolism rate, you have to understand what "metabolism" means.

The "official" definition of metabolism is "the process in which the body breaks down the fuel (proteins, carbohydrates, and fats) you eat and uses the products to generate the energy required for growth and life." In other words, metabolism is how efficiently (or fast) you use (or burn) energy (or calories). Now, hopefully that makes more sense!

The two main strategies for a more efficient metabolism are "MOVE IT" and "FUEL IT". A fitness combination of aerobic exercise and strength training burns calories and builds muscle, and the more muscle you have, the more calories you can burn. That's the MOVE IT part. But, if you do not feed your body the right kind of fuel at the right time, your muscles will run out of energy before they have reached their potential. Inadequate food, and even insufficient fluids, can slow down, even reverse, the benefits your body can gain from exercise. And that's the FUEL IT part! The two go hand in hand.

So it's a balance between food, fluid, and fitness. Maybe you know the food components of a healthy lifestyle, but just can't get your fitness plan in order. Or maybe you are consistent with your workouts, but the food and fluid components do not match your fitness efforts. It's a three-sided triangle, and if one side is out of balance, the other two sides will pay the consequences. But even if all three sides are in balance, if the foundation on which it rests is shaky, things will eventually fall apart.

Consider this: when a new car is under construction, the majority of the work effort is spent laying a strong foundation, making sure the engine, brakes, carburetor and all the intricate parts can support the functions of the car itself. Lots of effort, labor, and engineering skill are required to create a working model that will withstand the test of time and not be shaken by weather changes, daily wear and tear, and the inevitable aging process. These details are not visibly seen when the car is finally ready to go and on the lot; however, the ability of these "hidden" details to work together is what determines the success of the car's functions. So it is with your body's foundation, too. Your ability to read your body's hunger and fullness signals, the way your emotions support or sabotage your fitness efforts, and how you think about your body and its progress are all part of the foundation that can make or break your efforts.

Rev It Up! is designed to address the four "F's": Foundation, Food, Fluid, and Fitness, working together. Phase One (Weeks 1 through 4) presents weekly challenges for each of the four "F's", one for Food, one for Fluid, one for Foundation, and one for Fitness. You can choose to do just one or two challenges a week, but the program is designed to provide four weekly challenges that work together, with each week building on the previous week's progress. During Phase Two (Weeks 5 through 8), each week will focus on a single "F", like Foundation OR Fitness, to help you accelerate your progress. After completing both phases, Rev It Up! guides you through a maintenance plan (the rest of your life!) for your short and long term goals.

> *"I think the program really works because it's little changes every week instead of being overwhelmed by trying to make huge changes all at once."* Sabrina

You are encouraged to keep a journal in which you can write your specific daily goals, record your progress, and begin developing a strong, solid foundation to support your lifestyle changes. You may choose to write in the Maintenance Log, the journal pages starting on page 213 found in the back of this book-or simply use a blank notebook you already have on hand. Regardless of your choice, you will get the most out of this program if you journal regularly. As each week progresses, take a moment to summarize your progress on the "A Look in the Rearview Mirror" page located at the end of each week's lesson. These pages will help remind you of all the positive changes you have made, step by step, as you move through each phase of the program. Soon, you will be able to "hear" your engine running stronger, feel the difference it makes in your daily life and know that you are on your way to living well for a lifetime. So, ladies and gentlemen…..

START YOUR ENGINES!

Are You Ready to Rev It Up?

It is the mission of Rev It Up! to *"empower you to change from the inside out: find hope in your body's ability to change, feel confident in yourself and your body again, and live well-strong and balanced - through nutrition, fitness and behavioral modification education."* That sounds good, but not everyone may be ready to make the commitment to start living the Rev It Up! way.

Is Rev It Up! the right program, at the right time, for you? Only you can know for sure, so take this opportunity to assess *your* readiness for revving it up by answering the following questions:

1.   What other programs have you tried in the past?

2.   Which program worked best for you and why?

3.   On a scale of 1 to 10 (1= not at all, 10 = extremely important), how important is changing your eating/exercise habits to you?

4.   On a scale of 1 to 10, how confident are you in your capability to make the necessary changes?

5.   What is going on in your life right now that might "get in the way" of making changes in your lifestyle?

6.   List all of the positive benefits that you will receive by making healthy lifestyle changes.

7.   List all of the negative consequences that might occur by making healthy lifestyle changes.

8.   List all of the negative consequences that might occur by "staying the same".

9.   Do the positive benefits (Question #6) outweigh the negative consequences (Questions #7 and #8)?

Now take a moment to look over your responses. If your reasons for change, and commitment to do so, are based on the positive benefits you expect and your internal motivation to see the journey through, you are ready. If your willingness to make these changes in your current home and work environment is stronger than a 5 out of 10 (see Questions #3 and #4), then you are more than ready!

PHASE ONE:
Let's Get Started!

Week 1: Start Your Engine

Week 2: Move Your Car
Out of the Garage

Week 3: Get In Gear

Week 4: Tune Up

Week 1:

Start Your Engine

"Rev It Up! has changed my life! By losing the weight I did on this program so far, I had the proof I needed that I could lose weight by simply changing my eating habits. I always thought that to lose weight, one had to eat very little, no snacks between meals, give up the food I love, and never leave the gym. Thanks to Rev It Up!, I know that's not true! For the first time in my life while trying to lose weight, I am not always hungry or craving things I "can't" have. This program is something I know I can follow forever."   Mona

Chapter 1

Headlights on Foundation:
Check the Fuel Gauge

You are about to take the first step towards a Rev It Up! lifestyle-learning to communicate with your body. If you feel like your body is moving in one direction and you are moving in another, this is your opportunity to begin moving together. Your body is designed to do just that – to communicate with you so that you are going in the same direction. Your body can tell you when it needs fuel, but do you know how? How it tells you when it is running out? How it lets you know when it's had enough? If you are not sure, think about how your car communicates its need for fuel-the FUEL GAUGE.

How critical is your car's fuel gauge? If you have ever ignored the fuel gauge and ended up out of gas on the side of the road, you realize what important messages it sends, and how stressful it can be when you are not paying attention to the warning signs. The fuel gauge tells you when your gas tank is nearing empty and needs refueling. It also tells you when the gas tank is full and cannot hold any more without spilling out of the opening, wasting not only fuel but also money.

Just as important, your body's fuel gauge is the HUNGER and FULLNESS cycle. Hunger or fullness is how your body "talks" or communicates its needs for food and fluids. Do you pay attention to your body's fuel gauge or do you usually ignore or overlook its signals? Hunger tells you when your body is almost out of "gas" and needs refueling. Can you hear it, or do you wait for the yellow or orange panic light to come on or the beep to sound, and find yourself frantically searching for a quick fix, angry with yourself that you did not stop a few miles back when a gas station was convenient and you were not rushed? Fullness tells you when your tank is filled but not overflowing. Do you stop when you are full, or do you forget to pay attention and keep the fuel flowing in until it spills out, wasting your money and putting you and your car at risk?

Knowing *when* to eat and *when* to stop is the key to a truly "revved up" metabolism. When are you really hungry, and how hungry are you? At this point, you may be saying, "I don't even know what hunger feels like!" Maybe you have ignored the signals over the years, and now you no longer know how to "listen to" or read your fuel (hunger) gauge. Maybe you eat simply out of habit regardless of your body's need for fuel. Or you may have confused true physical, or stomach, hunger with "emotional" hunger needs. Are you really hungry for that chocolate candy bar on your way home from work? Or are you *emotionally* hungry for the comfort and stress relief that the chocolate candy bar provides?

Determining your *level of hunger* and the type of hunger takes time and practice, but the results are worth it. No other habit is more important to a lifelong change in the way you eat and the way you feel about what you eat. Knowing your hunger and fullness level allows you to work with and understand your body instead of feeling like you are "the last one to know" what your body really needs and, therefore, at the mercy of your food cravings. Being able to tell the difference between physical hunger and emotional hunger is a powerful tool that relieves you from food guilt and helps change your relationship with food from a constant battle to a trusting partnership.

So how do you begin learning how to read your fuel gauge? It starts with simply recording your hunger and fullness levels before and after you eat or drink. A scale from 1 (starving!) to 10 (stuffed!) is provided to help you learn to decipher your body's signals. At first this will feel awkward. Compare this to learning to drive a car using a gearshift system for the first time when all you have driven before is a car with an automatic transmission. The issue is not IF you can drive but HOW you drive.

If you have ever challenged yourself to learn how to shift gears, you remember that initially you had to concentrate constantly in order to shift to the right gear at the right time. You may have felt that the change was too difficult at first, but in a short time you were shifting gears easily and with confidence. A new habit was born through practice and concentration that expanded your driving potential.

Likewise, a new habit that will expand your own metabolism's potential is learning to know when and what to eat by listening to your body's communication signals, hunger, and fullness.

In the beginning, you may not be able to tell the difference between a "3" and a "7" and may record a "5" before and after every meal or snack. Don't give up! Little by little, you will begin noticing a change as you take the time to become more aware of your body's signals. And the emotional hunger will also begin to separate from the physical hunger so that you can "see" what your body really needs. This step is the most important Foundation challenge you will face. But the benefits are amazing: *The ability to control your food choices instead of food choices controlling YOU!*

The following list provides a hunger scale from 1 to 10. Use this list when you think about how hungry you are, and record that number in your Maintenance Log in the back of this book. If your Log isn't handy, simply jot it down anywhere. Don't think too much about your answer. Record what first comes to mind! Repeat this same procedure after you finish eating by choosing another number between 1 and 10 that signals how full you feel.

Your Hunger and Fullness Fuel Gauge: Scale of 1 (starving!)-10 (stuffed!)

1. You're dizzy and unable to think clearly. "I'm going to pass out if I don't eat right this minute!"
2. You're very irritable, and your stomach feels like an empty pit. Where IS that food...*any* food!?
3. You need to eat, but you aren't going to pass out... at least not yet!
4. You feel a little hungry, and your body is sending signals to fuel your engine.
5. Your stomach is in neutral. If you stop eating now, your fuel tank will need more fuel (food) in a few hours.
6. Your stomach knows that food has arrived, but you still want to eat a little more.

7. Your stomach is getting full now. If you stop eating, your fuel tank will not need more fuel, or food, until about 4 hours later.
8. You are full-that "deep, dark hole" has been filled to the top!
9. Your stomach is completely stretched to the point of discomfort, and one more mouthful may not even fit!
10. Help! Fuel overload! You really cannot eat even one more bite.

> *"The most beneficial part of Rev It Up has been*
> *learning to eat healthy without having to feel*
> *as if I was dieting, and understanding the process*
> *of when your body is hungry or full as (a guideline) to eat*
> *or not to eat. It is amazing how Rev It Up*
> *references our bodies needing food for fuel like a*
> *vehicle needs gasoline to run."*   Michelle

Your **FOUNDATION CHALLENGE** for Week 1: Before eating and/or drinking, stop and check your fuel gauge. How hungry are you before you eat? How full are you afterwards? **Record the level of hunger (H) and fullness (F)** in your Maintenance Log before and after each meal and snack. Begin noticing what your body is trying to tell you, look for any patterns of behavior and start to follow your body's lead.

Chapter 2

Headlights on Food:
Turn the Key

You have turned your headlights on your body's fuel gauge and taken a look at hunger and fullness. Now, it's time to turn on your body's engine! You know how to start your car's engine: simply put the key in the ignition and turn it! So how do you turn on your body's engine? Just as simple – fix BREAKFAST (the "key") and EAT it (the "turn" that starts the engine)! Breakfast is the meal that is most often ignored, but it is the most important. It's not called "break" the "fast" for nothing!

You may not feel that you have been "fasting", especially if you ate a second serving of dinner last night or lost control with a late-night snack before going to bed. You feel guilty, so maybe you should just skip breakfast. Surely your body can still find some fuel for this morning from your indulgences last night, right? Or maybe you just never eat breakfast because you don't wake up hungry. Or eating something in the morning makes you queasy. One meal cannot be that important, right?

Think again! Whatever fuel you put in your body the night before, it is either burned or stored by morning. As you sleep, your body is burning fuel to keep the heart pumping, blood circulating, lungs breathing, brain functioning-get the picture? Whatever fuel is available in excess, the body will store it (as fat) for future needs. So, your fuel tank is empty when you wake up even if you still feel full. What do you do?

You would not even think about backing your car out of the garage without first turning the key in the ignition. So why do you ask your body to "back out" and get moving, without starting its engine? Your fuel gauge is on empty in the morning, but your energy demands are increasing. You have about 1 to 1 ½ hours after getting out of bed to turn the key in the ignition and start the engine so that your car, or body, has fuel to move down the day's road. If you ignore the fuel gauge's "I'm on empty!" message, your body begins looking for other ways to take care of your fuel needs. It reacts to an empty fuel tank in ways that <u>protect</u> your body from burning fuel, since fuel is scarce. But do you really want your body protecting you from burning fuel, or calories? What your body does to help you store energy actually hurts you, and your metabolism, over time.

Let's look at what happens when you ignore your fuel gauge, do not eat, and your body feels threatened by the lack of available fuel, or calories, to meet the energy demands of your daily activities. Five changes begin to occur. The degree of change *varies* in every individual, and *depends* on how severe the restriction of energy (or calories) over time and how much activity is required. Regardless, all of the changes happen because your body is trying to take care of itself; however, the results end up hurting instead of helping your metabolism.

FIRST: Your body will start to <u>lower the rate it burns calories</u>, or fuel, to conserve as much energy as possible.

SECOND: Your body will begin to <u>protect its extra fuel stores</u>, your stored body fat, just in case you decide to skip the next meal, too. (Remember, it's not sure when you will fuel again!)

THIRD: Your body may <u>burn some of its own muscle tissue</u> for extra energy if burning less calories is not enough to make up for the lack of energy fuel. (Your own muscle tastes like chicken to an empty tank!)

FOURTH: Your body will trigger your brain to send signals to make LPL, or lipoprotein lipase. LPL is an enzyme that's main purpose is to <u>encourage your body to store fat</u>. More LPL in your body means more of the next meal's calories can be stored as fat instead of used immediately for energy.

FIFTH (and finally!): Your body will probably <u>crave fats and/or sugars</u> when it feels overdue for fuel: Fats, because this fuel group has the most calories per serving size, and sugar, because this fuel can be broken down very quickly. Who craves lettuce and carrots now? Don't be surprised if you cannot resist a quick drive through the fast food window!

At this point, your *willpower* is not the issue. Your fuel gauge has sent out its warning light, and your body has responded. It just so happens that its responses are geared to slow your metabolism instead of revving it up! So what can you do to start changing your body's response? Eat breakfast within 1 to 1 ½ hours after getting out of bed. It is as simple as that!

Do you already eat breakfast regularly, and within the right time frame? Good for you! And good FOR you! Did you know that regular breakfast eaters have less difficulty maintaining weight? Make healthier food choices throughout the rest of the day? Think clearer, and are more productive at work or school? Are less irritable when life throws a curve? If you fall into this category, you will find this week's Food Challenge easy. No problem, you can spend more time concentrating on the other challenges coming up! In the meantime, just keep eating breakfast, and record how hungry you are before, and how full you are after, you eat. Don't worry-you will learn more about what to eat, not only for breakfast but other meals, next week.

Caution Sign for Morning Exercisers

Do you exercise regularly in the early morning hours, and wonder how you can fit in breakfast? If you are an early bird that hits the gym or pavement before the sun comes up, simply plan on eating breakfast within 30 minutes AFTER finishing your workout. Eating within that 30-minute window is the ideal time for your muscles to recover this fuel level. This fuel helps re-fill the energy stores in your muscles so you are ready to go again the next morning. And if you are training for a competitive event, you may want to consider eating a small carbohydrate snack right before you work out to start the motor running, such as a banana, a small glass of juice or a handful of dry cereal. However, if weight loss is your goal, the pre-exercise snack may not be necessary.

However, most people find themselves in the category of a breakfast-skipper. It's time to look at some common excuses for not eating breakfast and decide to skip the excuses instead of the morning fuel! Do these sound familiar?

"I never really eat breakfast because I am never hungry when I wake up."

 Hmmm, you have just been challenged to "eat when hungry and stop when full". Since you aren't hungry in the mornings, wouldn't it be contradictory to eat? What's the deal?

Take a moment and imagine someone is trying to get your attention and calls your name repeatedly, but you ignore them, repeatedly. That person will eventually stop trying. Likewise, a body whose signals to eat have been ignored time and time again has probably learned to stop trying to get your attention. It will stay quiet, which means that your metabolism may stay asleep.   It will remain so until you decide to "wake it up" or turn it on by eating. If this is not until lunch, you have lost those hours that your body could be burning calories more efficiently. The body changes that result in a slower metabolism have started to occur because the fuel tank is empty yet the car, your body, has been asked to perform.

To break this negative cycle, a new pattern must be established. Eating something in the morning begins to re-activate your fuel gauge. As your body adjusts to having fuel available on an everyday basis, your metabolism adjusts, too. Instead of slowing down, it will begin to rev up since your gas tank is full! No more muscle being mistaken for chicken, less LPL enzymes running around waiting to store extra body fat, and fewer cravings that you cannot control. In other words, breakfast turns the key in the ignition, which starts the engine running, which starts fuel burning!

"I don't need breakfast in the mornings because I tend to overeat in the evenings, and therefore wake up feeling full, and guilty!"

You are nervous, because you know that you always overeat during the day, especially at night. Surely adding more food (calories!) at breakfast can only make matters worse, right? You have gained weight over time by not eating breakfast, so how will your body not gain even more weight if you add morning calories, too? Your concern is understandable. But, remember, NOT eating breakfast has not helped you maintain a desirable weight. It has not worked! It is time to change the way your body responds. Wake up your metabolism!

At first, eating something in the mornings may feel like you are just forcing calories in without eating any less through the rest of the day. And in fact, your evening meals may not be much smaller during the first week or two. Habits are hard to break! But remember that at least your body is arriving at that evening meal burning more calories during the day because you have eaten instead of skipped meals. As you continue concentrating on hunger and fullness signals, you will notice when a change begins.

You will stop eating out of habit and begin eating out of need. You will begin eating fewer calories in the evening because you do not like to feel a "10" on the fullness gauge-you are definitely no longer comfortable being that full! In turn, you will begin eating more during the day, and your energy level will take notice. Your meals will balance out as you begin to communicate with your body and use your fuel gauge. When your fuel tank is nearing empty again, you will be better able to listen and take action, choosing a healthier snack or meal instead of just whatever you can grab fast!

So no more excuses! If you are not a regular breakfast eater, start out simple and plain. Try a piece of whole-wheat toast with jam, or a cup of low-fat vanilla yogurt with fresh fruit, or a small bowl of cereal with low-fat milk. Remember to make a quick note of how hungry you are *before* eating, and then how full you are *after* eating. Watch for this to gradually change and improve, once your fuel gauge, or hunger cycle, starts matching up with your body's needs again. It's not being ignored any longer! And in about 3 weeks, you may notice that you wake up hungry for the first time in your life. That's a great sign of a metabolism that is up, burning calories, and ready to go!

"I was not a breakfast eater, but I have stuck with
the challenge of having breakfast within 1 ½ hours
of awakening. Just wanted you to know, for the first time

I was SO hungry for breakfast this morning! I can't ever remember being hungry for breakfast before!"   Sabrina

Your **FOOD CHALLENGE** for Week 1: **Eat breakfast within 1 to 1 ½ hours** after getting out of bed in order to turn on your car's engine and break the fast. In your Maintenance Log, record what you eat and drink, noting hunger (H) and fullness (F) levels before and after each meal.

WARNING: Your first week does NOT provide you with an easy way out! No list of specific breakfast meals from which to choose is given… just yet. You are being asked to concentrate on hunger and fullness levels, and how different food choices affect these levels. Do NOT proceed unless you want to begin making a difference in how you relate to your body. Do NOT proceed unless you want to begin experiencing control over your hunger and fullness levels. Do NOT proceed unless you truly want to gain ownership over your body and its weight changes. But if you DO, then keep going!

Chapter 3

Headlights on Fluid:
Watch Your Water Level

You may have heard that everyone needs a minimum of eight cups of water a day, but do you know where this originated? The amount of daily water you need is determined by how much daily water you lose. You lose water in your sweat, your urine, and even through breathing. To maintain water balance in your body, this fluid must be replaced. A general guideline is one liter of water (which is close to 1 quart, or 4 cups) for every 1000 calories you consume. If the average person consumes about 2000 calories every day, this translates to about 8 cups.

So do you need to actually drink this amount? Let's think about this a minute. Metabolism itself releases water back into your body-and can replace about 10% of your water losses. The foods you eat every day can replace about 20 to 40% of your water losses. So does this mean that you only need to drink up to 4 or 5 cups more? It IS true that metabolism of foods, and food itself, can give back about half of the water you lose every day. But you cannot stop there and assume that you only need 4 or 5 cups more until you look at the whole picture.

The typical American eats only 1 ½ servings of vegetables or fruits in any given day. Therefore, the foods that provide the most water are the least consumed. Furthermore, the typical American eats one out of every three meals at a sit-down or fast food restaurant and these meals are more processed and quite often much higher in sodium (or salt). Our bodies can function well on less than 2000 milligrams (mg) of sodium each day, but the average American eats two to four TIMES this amount, mostly from the processed or restaurant foods consumed. And it is a known fact that increased sodium in food increases fluid needs. So, your food choices have the potential to give back up to 40% of your water needs, but does today's lifestyle, with few fruits and vegetables and excessive amount of sodium, really include the foods that meet that need, on a daily basis?

What other factors influence your need for water? Your age helps determine fluid needs, since young children as well as older adults' needs are greater because they have less sensitivity to thirst and often become dehydrated. Your geographical location plays a part, since high altitudes or high humidity increase the need for more water. Your body size is a factor, because if you are overweight, your water needs are greater. And, if you choose to begin an exercise program, like you will in Rev It Up!, your water needs increase even more. The average American will typically only replace about 65% of the water lost in sweat if the decision is left up to perception of thirst only.

Let's keep looking at the role water plays in our health and our metabolism. Your body is about 60% water, and ALL energy reactions in your body, including the burning of fat calories, require water. Are you aware that water carries nutrients through the body and waste products out of the body? That water lubricates your joints to keep them moving? And water acts like a radiator to cool your body off when your temperature begins to rise, such as during exercise? And, finally, *more* water is the best solution when you are bloated? When the body gets less water than it needs, it senses this shortage as a threat and begins to hold on to every drop. The result? You feel, and are, bloated! Drink more water, and then your body will not feel threatened and will release the stored water it is holding.

Is water a factor in the process of metabolism itself? You bet! Water plays a role in the body's ability to metabolize, or burn, stored fat. Your kidneys cannot work properly without enough water. When they cannot carry their workload, they hand over some of their job responsibility to the liver. Since one of the liver's jobs is to turn stored body fat into energy that can be used (burned) by the body, the liver may have trouble operating at full speed if it has to do some of the kidney's work. If so, it may break down less fat, which means more fat remains stored in the body and weight loss potentially slows down. So, water keeps the kidneys working properly, which helps keep the liver doing its job of breaking down stored fat. So water has a role in the fat-burning process of metabolism.

Next benefit? Water helps maintain good muscle and skin tone. Did you know that water gives the muscle its natural ability to contract? A muscle that contracts is a muscle at work. A muscle at work means energy burned. Energy burned means your metabolism is revved up and doing its job! A "revved up" metabolism usually results in weight loss if your body is carrying more weight than it needs. Since weight loss can leave skin looking loose, water helps reduce this sagging by supporting your shrinking cells and keeping the skin plumped and healthy.

Last but not least, water can help remove waste produced when extra body fat is burned. So it would make sense that more water is needed to help flush out the extra waste caused by weight loss itself. Once again, it seems water is important for a more efficient metabolism and for optimal health.

But the real question comes down to this: What counts as "water"? What about those flavored or fitness waters? Can coffee count? Regular or decaffeinated? What about sodas – regular or diet? The Dietary Guidelines for Americans 2005 say that all of these fluids can hydrate because they all contain water; therefore, caffeine containing drinks can count towards your daily fluid needs.

What does Rev It Up! say? You will take a closer look at each one of these fluid options, including newer products like fitness or flavored waters, in Week 3. But for this week, if you are willing to take the Rev It Up! challenge *all the way*, let's try to stick with the tried and true fluid, water itself, to meet your first FLUID challenge.

Need some strategies to help you drink more water? Try one of these ideas:

1. "Don't leave home without it!" Keep a water bottle chilled and ready to go, and when you grab your car keys, grab a water bottle, too! Keep a water bottle in your car…and try to finish it off before you reach your destination. Fill it back up and drink more water on your way home.

2.   Purchase the 8-ounce individual bottles of water and put eight of these in your refrigerator as a reminder of your day's goal. You can "see" the full challenge, but it is in smaller increments. An 8-ounce portion may be easier to handle at one time than a big 24-ounce water bottle!

3.   Let a glass of water be the door that opens and closes a meal or snack. Before you begin eating, open the door by drinking 4 to 8 ounces of water. After you finish eating, close the door by drinking 4 to 8 ounces more.

4.   Add a little lemon or lime juice to give your water more pizzazz.

5.   Freeze a water bottle that is half full of water overnight. In the morning, fill up the remainder of the bottle with water. This will guarantee that your water stays cool for a longer period of time.

Your **FLUID CHALLENGE** for Week 1: Dive in and try to **double the amount of water you drink, up to 8 glasses a day**. If one glass is 8 ounces (or 1 cup), that's 64 ounces (or 8 cups) daily. In your Maintenance Log, check off one cup for every 8 ounces consumed.

Chapter 4

Headlights on Fitness:
Warm Up Your Motor

You have learned the "fuel it" strategies for the first week of Rev It Up!. Now it's time to use the fuel to "move it"! Think about your car again. It's no surprise that all the parts to your car are designed for movement-movement that's efficient and consistent to take you where you need to go.   Likewise, your body is designed for movement, too. Take a moment to remind yourself about all the benefits of moving your body.

How Does Exercise Benefit Your Body?

You may know that exercise can lower your blood cholesterol, reduce your blood pressure, strengthen your bones, and stabilize your blood sugar. Exercise may even help reduce your risk of developing diabetes and some types of cancer. And you know that exercise burns calories. What you may not know is that exercise actually improves your body's ability to burn stored body fat. Remember the enzyme LPL, whose job includes moving fat from your blood into fat cells for storage? Exercise counteracts LPL's fat-storing activity! It slows down LPL's activity in fat tissues, making it harder to store fat. And it increases LPL's ability to move fat into muscle cells so that it can be burned for energy instead of stored as more body fat. Sure, exercise burns calories, but it does so much more for you because it can literally change your fat-storing system into a more productive fat-burning system!

How Does Exercise Benefit Your Brain?

Exercise benefits your physical body in many ways, but it also benefits your *emotional* body. Many studies have shown that exercise not only increases your energy level but also helps relieve depression, improve self-esteem, and balance mood swings. Exercise triggers your brain to produce certain "feel good" chemicals called endorphins. These chemicals are related to the opium family and can produce a natural high that calms moods, lifts spirits, and improves self-confidence. With a stressful, fast-paced lifestyle, you need the emotional benefits alone that make regular exercise worth your time.

What Type of Exercise Do You Need To Do?

There are lots of reasons why moving your body is beneficial. But what kind of exercise is best? To rev up your metabolism, a combination of aerobic exercise and strength training is the goal. The first Fitness Challenge targets aerobic exercise, like walking, jogging, cycling or participating in a group exercise class like step aerobics. These types of exercise are called "aerobic" because you use a lot of "air", or oxygen, as you work. The key is to move your body in an activity that increases the number of heartbeats and the number of breaths you take per minute and keeps these numbers there for a steady period of time. And over time, your heart muscle grows stronger and larger, so that each beat is more efficient.

With more "powerful" heartbeats, the number of beats needed to do the same amount of exercise decreases. And your body learns to deliver oxygen to your muscles at a faster pace, so your heart does not have to work as hard since each beat is stronger and more oxygen is available to your working muscles. What a great tradeoff!

How Often and How Long Should You Exercise?

Of the two types of exercise, aerobic exercise should be done more often. Three times a week for 20 minutes each in your target heart rate range will help lower your risk of heart disease for sure, but to really rev up your metabolism, your body needs to exercise "more often than not." That translates to about 4 to 5 days each week. **Check with your doctor first** if you have not been physically active or have a medical history that might be affected by exercise. When you have your doctor's permission, start slowly and work up to 30 to 45 minutes each time at a pace that forces your heart to work harder.

**Caution Sign:
This is the Moment when the
Rubber Meets the Road!**

Stop and check out how you are feeling right now, at this very moment. Did you balk at reading the word "should"? Cringe at the mention of that "E" word (exercise) in general? Feel tired at the thought of 20 minutes, 3 days a week, let alone 30-45 minutes for 4 days a week?

In today's crazy-paced world, it's no wonder exercise can seem so difficult. How do you honestly fit it in? Is it worth it if you can only make time for 10 minutes a day, and not even every day? Especially when the calorie charts tell you that would only burn the equivalent of an apple? What if you literally hate to exercise? You do not even like to sweat?

These thoughts are real and can feel like permanent roadblocks. Sometimes it may be best to forget about the calories burned and the "I really should exercise" thinking. Start over, back at the beginning. The key is to begin a new *pattern*, even if it's just 10 minutes at first. Once the pattern of moving your body is set, it is easier to add more time later. So think about setting a new pattern of just moving more. Who knows where it might lead? Studies have shown that moving your body (exercise) has a healthy synergistic effect. Move your body regularly, and you actually begin choosing, better yet, desiring healthier foods. Consistent activity tends to change taste preferences from the typical high-fat fare to more lower-fat favorites. And that can happen without looking at a nutrition book or reading a calorie list!

If you are someone who struggles with even the thought of exercise, try one of these simple steps. Think small, set a pattern for this week's routine, and see if it doesn't begin changing your perspective!

1.   Concentrate on only the next 24 hours. Decide to take 10 to 15 minutes out of the entire 24-hour day to purposely move your body. (By the way, that leaves 23 hours and 45 minutes to do all your other routines!)

2.   Set clothes out the night before if getting up early to move, or if planning to move after work. Having a comfortable set of clothes ready to go, or already packed in the car, waiting for you to

leave your office, helps keep the pattern in place. Better yet, change at work – whether going to a gym, an outdoor track, even if going straight home. You will be ready to move when you walk into your own front door!

3.   Plan a distraction if you choose to move inside a gym or your home, such as on a treadmill. Read that magazine that came in the mail last week (most magazines can be read in about 10 to 15 minutes!). Read those journal articles stacked up on your desk. Choose five energetic songs and make a plan to move for those five songs only (five songs usually last about 15 minutes). Watch TV, or better yet, rent a movie DVD and play a 15-minute segment each time. If it is a really good movie, you will want to get back on that treadmill again just to see what happens next!

Now you have your body moving. One day planned at a time. A new pattern of lifestyle is in place. Feeling better now?

Is There Anything Else To Know?

Yes, there is-the **warm-up**. Take a minute and picture yourself getting in your car on a cold morning. You know you need to take a few minutes to allow your engine to warm up, so when you DO start driving, your car is ready to go and less likely to stall in the middle of traffic. Likewise, you also need to warm-up your body first. It may be easier to just jump into exercise-it saves you time, right? Well, eliminating the warm up may save a few minutes, at that moment, but you risk losing a lot of time later by decreasing your body's performance and increasing the risk of injury. An injury can put your body in the repair shop for a long time. Is it worth the risk?

Starting your activity ever so slowly allows your heart rate to increase slowly. It also helps change the direction of your blood flow away from organs like your stomach, where it is needed for digestion, towards your working muscles, for exercise. If you start moving too quickly without warming up, blood has to move VERY quickly to your muscles. This can not only make you nauseated because of the abrupt interruption of digestion but also rapidly increase your heart rate and your breathing. You will get tired more quickly, which cannot help but affect your desire to continue.

To warm up your muscles, allow for an extra 5 minutes to do the same activity but at a slower pace. For example, if you want to walk on the treadmill, warm up by starting out at a slower pace. Gently swing your arms by your side and very gradually increase the speed over 5 minutes. This plan works for ANY activity! The extra 5 minutes also give your mind a chance to relax, rid itself of the day's stress, and focus on your exercise goals.

Is That All?

"What goes up...must come down!" If the warm up is so important, so is the **cool-down.** Stopping abruptly stresses your muscles, and that includes your heart. It can increase your blood pressure, cause muscle cramps and soreness, make you dizzy, and increase your risk of injury. So always plan for some cool-down time, when you begin slowing down your pace and decreasing your heart rate-while you continue the same activity. Allow the cool down to gently take your muscles back to where they started so that they are ready to go again when YOU are!

The second part of a proper cool-down includes time to **stretch** those warm, flexible muscles! Exercise works your muscles, and during those contractions that you repeated over and over as you moved your body, your muscles have tightened. Tight muscles are shorter muscles. Stretching takes advantage of the warm muscle's flexibility, lengthening that same muscle, helping you relax, and improving your range of motion. This helps take away that soreness you may feel the next day, too.

Another reason? Stretching helps prevent the natural effect of aging! As you age, your muscles and joints lose flexibility, which may eventually affect your enjoyment of many daily activities. Stretching, done consistently, helps keep your muscles more flexible. And if your muscles are already warm from working out, you are able to receive the most benefit from each stretch.

Begin your stretches with the muscles you used the most. For example, if you walked, stretch the front and back of your thigh, and your calf muscles, first. Begin with the biggest muscles in that area and move to the smaller (i.e., thigh muscles before calf muscles). Next, stretch the upper body: torso, back, chest, shoulders, and arms, since they have helped balance and stabilize you during exercise.

Sample Stretching Routine

QUADRICEP (FRONT OF YOUR THIGH) STRETCH:
While holding a chair or other object for balance with your left hand, bend your right leg at the knee while bringing your right foot up behind you. Reach back with your *right hand and grasp the middle of your right foot or your right ankle. Your knee should be pointing straight down towards the floor and your hip should be relaxed. Do not lift your foot higher and pull your knee out of that straight down alignment. Remember to keep your opposite knee unlocked. Hold for 10 to 15 seconds and repeat on opposite side. You should feel this stretch in the front muscles of your thigh. For a more advanced stretch, let go of your stabilizing chair or wall and lift the opposite arm (from the leg being stretched) out to the side so that you add some benefit to the balancing muscles during your stretch.

*People with knee trouble may wish to use the opposite hand and reach behind the back to grasp the foot of the bending leg in order to protect the knee from possible injury.

HAMSTRING (BACK OF YOUR THIGH) STRETCH:
Place your right foot on a chair or elevated object that is lower than your hips. Do not lock your knee. Gently "sink" into the stretch by bending the opposite knee and lowering your body. Hold for 10 to 15 seconds, and repeat with the opposite leg.

CALF STRETCH:
Facing a wall, press your right foot against the wall, keeping your heel stationary against the floor and a slight bend in your knee. Hold for 10 to 15 seconds and repeat with your opposite foot.

TORSO:

Stand with feet hip width apart and slowly lift straightened arms out in front of you until they are reaching straight up and your elbows are just in front of your ears. Hands should be open with palms facing inward. Take a deep breath and as you exhale, slowly bend to the right and hold while you take slow, deep breaths for 10 to 15 seconds. Return to center and stretch upward for 10 to 15 seconds. Repeat to the left side.

CHEST STRETCH:

Clasp your hands behind your back. Extend your arms up and out, as if you are trying to pull your shoulder blades together. Hold for 10 to 15 seconds.

BACK STRETCH:

Clasp your hands in front of your chest, arms extended. Reach forward as if you are pulling your shoulder blades apart. Hold for 10 to 15 seconds.

SHOULDER STRETCH:

Stand up straight and tall. Bring your right arm across your chest, supporting with your left hand. Feel the stretch in your right shoulder. Consciously drop, or relax, the right shoulder even more if you can. Hold for 10 to 20 seconds, and repeat with other arm.

There are many more stretches you can do, but these target the major muscles and will help you begin a routine that will keep you flexible and help prevent injuries down the road. Remember to breathe deeply and slowly during each stretch!

The "Anything Else?" is definitely "something else," isn't it? *A warm-up, AND a cool-down including good stretch time.* Can you still keep your workout commitment to an amount of time that is realistic? Sure! A 5-minute warm-up can be followed by 30 minutes of aerobic exercise and concluded with 10 minutes to cool down and stretch. So, yes, you can. The big question: Is it worth it? Absolutely! It's an investment in your body's ability to KEEP on exercising!

Your **FITNESS CHALLENGE** for Week 1: **Choose an aerobic activity you enjoy, and commit to move your body (with your physician's permission).** If you are new or just resistant to regular body movement, start small with simple goals. Get a new lifestyle *pattern* set. You can add to your pattern as the weeks pass, but try to commit to include a warm-up AND cool-down each time. It doesn't really matter what time of day you choose-if you are not a morning person, do not plan to attend a 5:30am aerobics class! Find a time that works with your schedule-and commit to moving your body, consistently, with a long-term goal of 4 days out of every week. Use your Maintenance Log to record your progress (what you do, when you do it, and for how long).

A Look in the Rearview Mirror

Week 1: Start Your Engine

Foundation: Before eating or drinking, stop and check your fuel gauge. Record the level of hunger (H) and fullness (F) in your Maintenance Log before and after each meal and snack.

Food: Turn the key by eating breakfast every morning within 1-1 ½ hours after rising.

Fluid: Dive in and try to double the amount of water you drink, up to eight glasses daily.

Fitness: Choose an aerobic activity you enjoy, and commit to move your body (with your physician's permission), working up to four different days. Gradually work up to 45 to 60 total minutes, which includes warm-up and cool-down.

Record any changes you notice this week:

Date	Thoughts, Feelings, Body Changes?

Week 2:

Move Your Car
Out of the Garage

"With all the gimmick and fad diets out there, this is actually a wellness program that doesn't make me feel deprived or that I'm on a diet. This may seem like a small thing, but it's been the most important: using 'ping pong ball' portions from the fat group and using the size of my hand as a guide to the right size in meat or protein portions. That helps keep me on a healthy track."   A.R.

Chapter 5

Headlights on Foundation: Align Your Fuel Timing

You are on your way to building a new foundation by checking your fuel gauge, or your hunger/fullness levels, before and after each meal or snack. The next Foundation strategy for a revved up metabolism that goes hand-in-hand with your fuel gauge is the alignment, or balance, of meals and snacks. In past attempts to lose weight, have you tried to balance the amount of fuel (*what* you eat and drink) but ignored the need to balance the timing (*when* you eat and drink)? The "what" and "when" are both important steps to moving on out!

Let's start with the "when". To turn the key in the ignition, you have started eating breakfast within 1 to 1 ½ hours after getting out of bed. Now, let's take it one step further and align the rest of your meals and snacks to keep your engine fueled throughout the entire day.

Think back to your car again. You know it's time to fuel your car when you see the needle on your fuel gauge nearing the empty level, right? Most cars are equipped with reminders to warn of a low gas tank-either a light appears or a beep is heard. Some even have a programmed voice telling you fuel is needed. Wouldn't it be nice if our bodies had the same clear warning features?

If you are paying attention, you hear the warning before you reach empty, stop, and fill your gas tank. Sometimes you may accidentally find yourself on empty without realizing it because you ignored the signals or did not stop long enough to notice. In more of a panic now, you quickly rush to find a gas station, hoping you make it before you run out of fuel. Often you will not have the time to locate the best price or your favorite brand-you're just lucky to find anything and find it fast!

Once at the pump, it makes sense to go ahead and fill the fuel tank completely. Saves you time in the long run. But occasionally you may have to put in just a few dollars-maybe that's all the cash you have available or you don't have enough time to fuel the entire engine at that moment. The extra few gallons of fuel will give you the boost you need to buy some time until you have an opportunity to fill it up.

How do you know when your tank is full? The nozzle clicks off, right? (if only our bodies were that easy!) Even if you are on a long trip to one of your favorite destinations and know that you have hours to go before you are there, you still cannot add any more fuel once the tank is full. Well, you *could* override the pump and force more fuel into the tank, but the gas has nowhere left to go. It spills out, on to the car, down to the ground, and is completely wasted. Or you could buy the extra tank of gas and store it in a container, but you still would have to wait to use it, and storing gas in a moving car has its consequences! Whichever the circumstance, the gas cannot be used then, but you still have to pay for it, right?

"I would never overfill my tank like that and waste gas and money!" Yes, you are right. You *do* know your tank's limitations and how to meet your car's fuel needs depending on your daily plans. But do you know that much about your own body, and how to meet its fuel needs without overflowing?

Pumping gas into a fuel tank is like fueling your metabolism with regular stops at mealtimes. Let's compare the two:

Your body's fuel tank holds about 4 hours worth of fuel at any given time. Your fuel gauge is your hunger and fullness cycle. As your hunger approaches a 3 out of a 10 on the hunger scale, your body's warning light, hunger, lets you know that it's time to look for fuel. Ideally you have some time to look around and find the best price and brand of "fuel" (food) for your "car"(body), either at a restaurant or at home. When you find it, you stop, fill up the tank by eating a meal, and hit the road again, fueled and ready.

As the day continues, you notice your hunger is approaching a 3 out of 10 again. You have several commitments and know it's going to be a few more hours before your next meal, so you stop and refuel with a snack, or a few dollars worth of fuel to buy some time until you can fill it up.

What if you don't pay attention to your hunger cycles, and you realize you are a 1 out of a 10 before you had a chance to look for the nearest fuel (food) station? You will be very quick to choose something fast and easy, regardless if it is the best choice in health and price or not. Fast food restaurants or convenience store snacks become too hard to pass up when you are out of fuel and out of time!

Or maybe you know you are going to your favorite restaurant for dinner. So you plan to skip your lunch so you can eat more calories at dinner without feeling guilty. *Not a good idea!* First of all, you will be so hungry that your cravings will increase and your ability to make healthy, balanced choices will be compromised. Secondly, it is inevitable that you will overeat at that meal. That is no different from standing at the pump with your hand holding the lever down as gas continues to flow even after the nozzle clicks and the pump reads full. You keep filling beyond the amount that your tank can hold. This wastes calories and ends up inevitably being wasted and stored as body fat. *Somehow it is a lot easier to see the consequences of over-fueling your gas tank than it is over-fueling your body's tank.*

The important lesson here is meal timing! So follow these simple guidelines:

1) Breakfast needs to be eaten within 1 to 1 ½ hours of getting up and going (You are doing this already, right?).

2) All other meals or snacks need to be eaten within 4 hours of the previous meal or snack. *Example A*: You ate breakfast at 6:30 a.m. and lunchtime will not arrive until around noon, so you eat a snack at about 10 a.m. to keep your engine fueled! *Example B*: You ate breakfast around 8:00 a.m., so you will not need to eat a morning snack since your lunch break is at noon. But plan ahead for that long afternoon stretch! *Example C*: You eat lunch at noon, but dinner is not planned until after 6:00p.m. Therefore, an afternoon snack around 3:00 p.m. will be necessary to keep

your engine running efficiently and prevent cravings before dinner.

3) What about snacks *after* dinner? Late-evening snacks are not mandatory and probably not necessary for most people. Your body will begin slowing down in its preparation for sleep and does not need any additional energy. But, in certain situations, an after-dinner snack may be necessary if you are going to remain active for a long period of time after your dinner meal. *Example A*: You are a student staying up late to study for an exam. You had dinner at 6 p.m. and it is already 10 p.m., and you are not finished. A snack is probably a good idea to keep you energized to continue studying and to prevent that late-night refrigerator raid! *Example B*: You are a business person and up late completing a project. Yes, the same suggestion applies to you. Do not be afraid of eating later in the evening if you are busy with work or an event and you find yourself hungry again after 3 or 4 hours have passed since dinner. But, if you are just sitting and watching the evening news before you go to bed, your body does not need an energy boost. There is no hard and fast rule that prohibits evening snacking-listen to your body, check out the situation, and respond according to your needs. But if weight loss is your goal, be cautious about fueling your tank when your car is parked in the garage!

So, that is how you take the next step to align your meals and snacks. You have already started eating breakfast. Now just watch the clock and make sure that you fuel your engine within 4 hours of each meal or snack. As the availability of fuel stays consistent, you will notice that your hunger, or fuel gauge, begins to match up to the clock. And as you become more aware of your hunger and fullness levels, you will not need to watch the clock-you will simply be able to listen to your body and respond to your brain's signal to eat.

Do you hear yourself saying, *"I just don't know about this? You tell me to follow my hunger signals but then you ask me to eat every 4hours. I am NOT hungry every4 hours! What gives?"* Initially, you may feel that you are a slave to Father Time, having to eat based on a clock without feeling or knowing you are really hungry. And if you have always eaten a big dinner meal, you may not quickly decrease the quantity at that meal just because you've eaten more throughout the day. Habits are difficult to break! But don't forget several truths:

1. If you have eaten more throughout the day, your body will arrive at that dinner meal burning more calories than it used to burn at that time.
2. You will have a well-fueled, clear mind so that you can make conscious decisions about how much and what to eat.
3. Gradually, but consistently, your three meals will begin lining up so that each meal is no bigger or smaller than the other.
4. Because you are now eating from hunger and fullness signals, you will notice that you are not as hungry and will begin eating less at dinner based on your own decision.,
5. At this point, you OWN your body changes! Congratulations!

If these five reasons do not provide enough assurance, try this. Repeat the following four-word sentence, with confidence, when you feel the need to keep eating even though you know you are not really hungry anymore: **I CAN EAT AGAIN!**

Now repeat it again, emphasizing the first word: **I** can eat again. Now the second word: I **CAN** eat again. Then the third word: I can **EAT** again. Finally the fourth word: I can eat **AGAIN**. There is something strangely comforting about saying "I can eat again!" You may know it intellectually but do your actions often reflect something different? Somehow it's easier to eat each meal as if it is the last, rather than be willing to put the fork down when your fuel tank is full but the rest of the lasagna is still sitting on your plate, or the last half of that slice of pie is calling your name.

No one is telling you not to have it, but just have it later, when your fuel tank actually needs more fuel. Then the body can and will use it, not when it overflows from a tank that is already full but when it flows into a tank that is empty and ready for more!

Once you align the timing of your meals and snacks, you may start to notice that your cravings begin to lessen. This may be most apparent in the afternoon if you have never stopped to eat a snack even though your lunch and dinner are always more than 4 hours apart. When your body is fueled consistently, and is not allowed to get too hungry between meals, the cravings for fats and sugars begin to disappear. Isn't that a wonderful benefit of eating a snack?

If that is not enough, keep an eye on changes in your energy level, too. With consistent fuel, you will see your energy level become more consistent. And you will feel better! Both energy increases and craving decreases are evidence of a changing metabolism. You are on your way!

> *"I really feel that I know so much more about my body now than ever, and feel 100% better than I have felt for years. I know part of it is because I know I look better but much of it is that I have so much more energy. Tonight I actually crossed my left leg over my right one, and I cannot tell you how long it has been since I did that comfortably."* Doris

Your **FOUNDATION CHALLENGE** for Week 2: Eat breakfast within 1 to 1 1/2 hours after rising, and **do not wait longer than 4 hours between each meal or snack.** Record the times you eat in your Maintenance Log.

Chapter 6

Headlights on Food:
Balance Your Fuel Content

See how it all begins to work together? Now let's examine the other important step to meal alignment-the "WHAT":

A.   A balanced meal needs to include 3 to 4 fuel (food) groups to qualify.
B.   A balanced snack needs to include 1 to 2 fuel (food) groups to qualify.

What exactly is a fuel group? Although more than 40 different nutrients with many different functions are required for good health, these nutrients can be divided into just five food groups-all of which provide fuel for your body. Hence the term, fuel group! One single fuel group is not more important than another because each group has different "jobs" or priorities in the body. Our body is an amazing machine that requires fuel from all the food groups to produce its best work. And these same fuel groups can be divided into those that provide ENERGY (to specifically fuel the brain and all your body's functions and movement) and those that provide PROTEIN (for replacing and building cells, hormones, enzymes, and muscles among other jobs!) The five fuel groups that you will use to build a meal or snack include the *energy* fuel groups: Grains and Starches, Fruits and Vegetables, and the *protein* fuel groups: Animal/Plant Proteins and Dairy Proteins.

You need both energy and protein at all three meals-breakfast, lunch and dinner. For snacks, it depends on the time frame. If you have just an hour or so before lunch, a mid-morning snack for only energy gives you that little boost you need. But since you usually need more fuel in the afternoon to break the six or more hour time span between lunch and dinner, your afternoon snack needs both energy and protein from two fuel groups. Protein, when eaten with an energy fuel, helps make the energy from that grain or fruit or vegetable last longer, and also helps prevent cravings. Therefore, energy and protein fuels work together-whether eaten at meals or snacks-to provide more lasting energy and a healthier balance of fuel.

A complete table of what foods go into each fuel group is right around the corner, but before you read any further about what to eat, you may have already noticed that certain well-loved foods have not been mentioned yet. Are you asking yourself, "Where are those desserts hiding? What about a glass of wine? And I don't see any French fries!" Indeed they have not been mentioned specifically yet, but do not panic! These "other" foods do have a place, but the other fuel group is just that-OTHER. It does not count as one of the fuel groups from which to build a meal or snack. The "other" foods simply *complement* your meals and snacks. So look at how to build a meal or snack from the five basic fuel groups first, then you will discover how the "other" group fits in.

Are you ready to learn how to build a meal? You will need to remember the following guidelines:

A MEAL = 3 to 4 fuel groups (for both energy and protein)

A SNACK = 1 to 2 fuel groups (depends on time of day)

    Mid-morning snack = 1 fuel group for energy only

    Mid-afternoon snack = 2 fuel groups for energy and protein

Next, you will need to know how much a portion is for each fuel group. Does this mean you have to weigh and measure your foods? No! Does this mean that you have to keep a food reference handy that lists portions and calories for each food? No! So, what does this mean for you, someone who desires to lose weight but needs a road map that guides your path without becoming unrealistic, demanding, or complicated?

In Rev It Up! terms, you'll need only three simple tools to keep you on the right road: a baseball, a ping pong ball, and the palm of your hand. Breathe a sigh of relief and throw out that old calorie-counting book! Toss the fat gram counter! For a reference, study the following:

1. A **baseball** is approximately 2.94" wide:

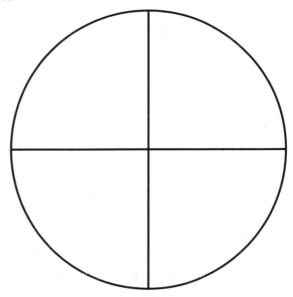

2. The **palm of your hand**…you should have one of these with you!

3. A **ping pong ball** is approximately 1 ½ " wide:

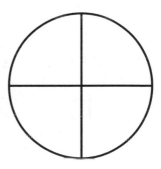

Now take a closer look at each of these:

Visualize a baseball on your plate. Technically, you could cut a baseball in two and fill each side with mashed potatoes-and both sides would equal one full cup (It's true!). However, "technical" does not always represent "realistic." Who carries around a measuring cup and levels off a serving perfectly? And if you had to technically represent a true serving of every grain or starch, fruit or vegetable, the differences can vary from a tennis ball to a softball size, depending on the density of the food you are measuring. So, stay simple and realistic. Think baseball circumference, and count one-half baseball as roughly the size of 1 portion of grain or starch, and one baseball as roughly the size of 1 portion of fruit, vegetable or soft dairy protein like cottage cheese. (Other liquid-based dairy products, like yogurt or milk, still need the typical 8-ounce or 1-cup portion).

The palm of your hand is the amount of protein you need at each lunch and dinner. A palm is usually about 3 to 5 ounces, depending on the bone structure and size of the person; therefore, a large-boned, taller person will need more protein than a small-build, petite person. Your palm answers the question for lunch and dinner, but what about breakfast? Typically the size of half of your palm is equal to one egg, for women, and two eggs, for men. It's doubtful you will eat, or even need, eggs every day, which is why the breakfast meal proteins are unique. Dairy products, even nuts and seeds, fit well at breakfast, too. Answers to more of your breakfast questions can be found shortly when you look at examples of breakfast meals.

A ping pong ball is roughly the size of 1 portion of snack proteins, like peanut butter (1 tablespoon = 1 ping pong ball), nuts/seeds (1 tablespoon= 1 ping pong ball) or block-style cheese (1 ounce "block" = 1 ping pong ball). A ping pong ball is also about the size of 1 portion (1 tablespoon) of fat, like salad dressing, mayonnaise, butter, margarine, sour cream, cream cheese, oil…in other words, the fats you add to foods to increase flavor and texture. Again, think ping pong ball *circumference*. Nuts certainly vary in size, and peanut butter is denser than vegetable oil, so "technically" a serving might vary between a large marble and a golf ball. But stay simple, and realistic, and count one ping pong ball as roughly 1 portion of snack proteins and 1 portion of higher-fat condiments.

Overwhelmed? Take a slow, deep breath and repeat: "I solemnly swear that I will NOT panic until I have read through this entire chapter." You will see how it all works together in just a few minutes. Right now, simply read each fuel group that follows, and note the recommended portions for each, depending on if it's a meal or a snack. *Please note:* Portion guidelines are specific for general weight loss and may need to be individualized. See a registered dietitian for a more individualized plan if needed.

ENERGY FUEL GROUP	PORTION GUIDELINES FOR WEIGHT LOSS
GRAINS and STARCHES (WHOLE GRAIN OR 100% WHOLE-WHEAT preferred) • Breads, including pita, bagels, tortillas, roll/bun • Beans/peas, like lentils, navy, pinto, lima, garbanzo • Corn, including tortillas and popcorn • Crackers • Oats and cereals, hot or cold • Pastas • Potatoes, white and sweet • Pretzels, low-fat chips • Rice, brown preferred	For **meal**: 1baseball (*women*) or 1 ½- baseballs (*men*) For **snack***: 0- ½ baseball (*women*) or 0-1 baseball (*men*) (*"0" means you can choose another energy fuel like vegetable or fruit for a snack instead of choosing a grain) Note: 1 bread slice/roll = ½ baseball

ENERGY FUEL GROUP	PORTION GUIDELINES FOR WEIGHT LOSS
FRUITS • All fresh fruits • All canned fruits, NO sugar added • All frozen fruits, NO sugar added • All dried fruits*, NO sugar added	For **meal** or **snack** (*women and men*): 1 baseball *2 ping pong balls for dried fruits

ENERGY FUEL GROUP	PORTION GUIDELINES FOR WEIGHT LOSS
VEGETABLES • All fresh vegetables • All frozen vegetables, without cream sauces (Canned vegetables are not preferred due to high level of sodium and low level of fiber)	For **meal** or **snack** (*women and men*): 1or more baseballs

PROTEIN FUEL GROUP	PORTION GUIDELINES FOR WEIGHT LOSS
DAIRY PROTEINS • Cheeses, part skim or 2% milk based preferred • Cottage cheese, 1% • Milk, fat free or 1% • Yogurt, fat free or 1% Try to include at least 2 servings (*men*) or 3 servings (*women*)* of dairy daily to get the calcium needed to maintain strong bones.	For **meal** or **snack** (*women* and *men*): 1 ping pong ball of cheese (block style, or 1 slice prepackaged) 1 baseball of cottage cheese 1 cup (8 ounce) yogurt or milk *If you do not include this amount consistently, consider taking a calcium supplement with Vitamin D.

PROTEIN FUEL GROUP	PORTION GUIDELINES FOR WEIGHT LOSS
ANIMAL / PLANT PROTEINS **Animal Proteins:** • Beef, lean cuts preferred • Canadian bacon • Deli sliced meats, lean • Egg or egg substitutes (Continued on next page)	For **breakfast meal** (*women and men*): 1/2 palm size (Example: 1 egg for women, two for men) For **lunch and dinner meals** (*women and men*): palm size

• Fish, fresh, frozen, canned • Pork, lean cuts preferred • Poultry, without skin **Plant Proteins:** • Beans/lentils (NOTE: These are also grain fuels.) • Soy products, including tofu • Vegetarian meats	For **lunch and dinner meals** (*women and men*): palm size
Snack Proteins: • Peanut butter, natural preferred • Nuts and seeds	For **snack** (*women and men*): 1 ping pong ball Note: These plant proteins are best for snacks because of the higher calorie content.

*[As stated, these recommendations are **for weight loss** for most individuals. Discuss these guidelines with a registered dietitian if you feel they do not meet your specific needs or circumstances. If your goal is **sports performance**, you will need to increase the recommended number of servings depending on your exercise level.]*

So all you need is a baseball, a ping pong ball, and the palm of your hand. Can it really be that simple? Yes! Each day is different, and hopefully you eat a variety of grains, fruits, and vegetables for your energy fuel, and a variety of animal, plant, and dairy proteins. It will all balance out in the long run, but only having three real-life objects as portion guides make it simple. You can go anywhere and keep your portions in control, without a calorie guidebook or fat gram counter, when you visualize a baseball or your palm as your guide. Likewise for a ping pong ball!

Is it time for another deep breath? All of this discussion about energy fuel, protein fuel, and portion guidelines can seem overwhelming at first, especially if you are used to receiving simple lists of "correct" foods to eat with specific measurements or recipes for each. A long list of "good and bad" foods is certainly easier in some ways-especially initially-because you do not have to think too hard to follow the plan. But is it realistic? What if you don't *like* most of the foods on the "good" list-what do you choose then? What if you make a mistake and eat the "wrong" thing? You have failed the plan and feel like giving up instead of embracing the opportunity to learn how your body's fuel gauge responds to different types of fuel. And what happens when you get tired of that list-how do you maintain control over your weight then?

OWNERSHIP of the changes your body makes-whether it is in weight loss, increased energy or decreased cravings-is so important. An easy "good and bad" food list takes the ownership away from YOU, and any success achieved is usually temporary. So you quit. But when you want to lose weight again, you pick up the list and try again. The problem? You have not changed the patterns and habits that got you there in the first place. Ownership of your food choices leads to ownership of your body's successes-that truly makes the long term difference!

Let's talk through another example. When you are looking at a map to a new city, many different choices exist, and the route you choose will depend on your priorities. Do you want to take the scenic route, or do you need to take the interstates in order to save time? It's up to you. Regardless of your reasons, you have to study the map to find the route that works best for you. And, inevitably, you might make a few wrong turns, but you realize your mistake when the landmarks you are passing do not match up to the ones you expect. Your unexpected detour slows you down, but it also makes you pay more attention. And you will probably not make the same mistake again since you are more focused now!

But if someone is driving *for* you, your responsibilities change dramatically. It's doubtful that you will pay attention to the roads you are traveling, since riding as a passenger is much easier and requires little concentration on your part. This works well for you as long as the driver is available-but what happens if you are required to drive yourself the next time? You have no one to depend on but yourself to find your way back home, but you don't know the right way to go. You did not pay attention to the turns that you needed to make and now you find yourself lost and confused about what direction to take.

If you know that feeling of being frustrated with yourself when you cannot remember simple turns, get lost, and waste valuable time in the process, then you can hopefully relate to how it feels if you have been following a "good and bad" food list, without having to think, until all of a sudden it's not working for you anymore. The diet is over, the list is gone, and you are on your own. You find yourself going in circles, or just going back the way you came and giving up. A diet that tells you exactly what food to eat at every meal is just like someone driving *for* you. Ownership of your body is following guidelines but having to make your own food choices, some good and some bad. Ownership of your body is learning from every good and not so good choice and feeling more confident as you get closer to your goal.   And as you own your mistakes as well as your progress, you can take 100% credit for your inevitable success!

Convinced that you want to give this ownership thing a try? Great! Let's put the Rev It Up! guidelines together and see how it works. At each meal-breakfast, lunch and dinner-you need both energy and protein-from 3 to 4 fuel group choices. At each snack, which is designed to give you a few extra "miles" before you stop for a fill-up, you need less fuel than at your meal times, so select only 1 to 2 fuel group choices. At your morning snack, you probably need just energy (1 fuel group) unless you work out in the early morning, then you can consider adding protein, too. At your afternoon snack, you definitely need energy and protein (2 fuel groups).

How about some examples of different meals and snacks using the different fuel groups? Check out the following ideas:

Breakfast Examples:

An example of a balanced breakfast, using 3 fuel groups, is cold cereal like Raisin Bran (amount of 1baseball for women, 2 for men), small grapefruit (1 baseball), and 1% milk (1 cup).

3 fuel groups = GRAIN (cereal) + FRUIT (grapefruit)
+ DAIRY (milk)

Did this provide both energy and protein? Yes! Energy from the grain and fruit, and protein from the milk. A good example of a balanced meal providing energy and protein that meets the 3 to 4 fuel group goal. A second example, using 4 fuel groups, is a toasted English muffin (2 halves for women, 3 halves for men), served "sandwich style" with slices of tomato (amount of 1 baseball), a scrambled egg or two (1/2 to 1palm size portion) and reduced-fat (2% milk) cheese (1 individual slice).

> 4 fuel groups = GRAIN (muffin) + VEGETABLE (tomato)
> + ANIMAL PROTEIN (egg) + DAIRY (cheese)

Did this meal provide energy and protein? Yes, energy from the grain and vegetable, and protein from the egg and cheese. A balanced meal providing energy and protein that meets the 4 fuel group goals. If you were wondering how a vegetable could fit at breakfast, you can see that tomatoes or other choices like bell peppers, mushrooms, and onions work great! You can even sauté them, adding them to your scrambled egg for variety.

Lunch or Dinner Examples:

An example of a balanced lunch or dinner is a whole-wheat pita pocket (1 pita for women, 1 ½ - 2 for men) stuffed with deli-sliced turkey (palm-size portion), lettuce shreds and tomato slices (at least 1 baseball), with strawberries (1 baseball) on the side.

> 4 fuel groups = GRAIN (pita) + VEGETABLE (lettuce/tomato)
> + FRUIT (strawberries) + ANIMAL PROTEIN (turkey)

A second example: How about a grilled pork tenderloin (palm size portion) with steamed asparagus (at least 1 baseball), a small baked sweet potato (size of 1/2 baseball for women, 1 baseball for men), and a whole grain roll (1/2 baseball)?

> 3 fuel groups = GRAIN (sweet potato and roll) + VEGETABLE
> (asparagus) + ANIMAL PROTEIN (pork)

You can add a ping pong ball-sized amount of butter or margarine to flavor your potato and roll. More on those OTHER foods coming up soon!

If you prefer combination type foods, a third example is thin crust vegetable pizza. The crust is your grain (1 baseball = 2 slices thin crust for women, 3 for men), the cheese (about 1 ping pong ball per average pizza slice) is your dairy, and the vegetables (hopefully enough for 1 baseball amount) speak for themselves! Adding a side salad (another baseball) with "light" vinaigrette dressing (up to 1 ping pong ball amount) will top it off.

3 fuel groups = GRAIN (pizza crust) + VEGETABLE (tomato sauce
with vegetable toppings, salad) + DAIRY (cheese)

Snack Examples:

A "1 fuel group" snack, ideal for a midmorning pick-up, can be graham crackers (1/2 baseball = one large rectangle, or 2 "squares") *or* an apple (one baseball). Carrot sticks (one baseball) can certainly fit as well. The grain, fruit or vegetable fuel groups provide the energy you need for that midmorning boost. A dairy fuel, like one cup of low fat (1%) yogurt or milk, also fits well.

1 fuel group = GRAIN *or* FRUIT *or* VEGETABLE *or* DAIRY

A "2 fuel group" snack, ideal for the afternoon stretch when dinner will be much later, can be whole-wheat crackers (1/2 baseball amount equals 6 to 8 crackers) and a mozzarella cheese stick (about 1 ping pong ball). Another example is low-fat vanilla yogurt (1 cup, or 8 ounces) with banana slices (1 baseball) added. How about apple slices (1 baseball) with peanut butter (1 ping pong ball amount)? Or even whole grain cereal (1/2 to 1 baseball size amount) and 1% milk (1 cup or 8 ounces)?

2 fuel groups = GRAIN + DAIRY *or* FRUIT + DAIRY *or*
FRUIT + PLANT PROTEIN

Other snack examples will be provided soon. But in the meantime, hopefully this helps you see how you can build a meal or snack, using the fuel groups to enjoy lots of variety while keeping your metabolism boosted! Even though giving a list of ready-to-go snack choices would be easier to follow, it takes away from your ownership of what you decide to eat. The list is purposefully delayed until Chapter 14 (Week 4) so that you can experiment with your own combinations and use your own hunger and fullness signals to decide what works for you or doesn't. The same principle holds true for meals, too. A ready-to-go list of lunch and dinner choices is easier but takes away the learning process. Remember, you want to drive the car, not be the passenger! It's all about ownership! Why don't you take a turn building sample meals and snacks? Fill in the following table, using some of your favorite foods:

Type of Meal	Fuel Choices	Portion Guide	# of Fuel Groups	Correct Portions
BREAKFAST				
LUNCH				
DINNER				
SNACK				

How did you do? Were your meals 3 to 4 fuel groups? Snacks 1 to 2? How did you estimate your portions (remember, baseball, ping pong ball, and palm of your hand!)?

Do you have to pre-plan your meals like this? No, but now you know you can if you need or want to do so!

Some of the examples above used fuel from the "Other" fuel group to complement the meal. It's time now to look at what foods fall into this "Other" group. The following table lists these foods for you; however, since these foods have lots of calories and few, if any, nutrients, react to these foods as you would react in any high-traffic area:

PROCEED WITH CAUTION!

THE "OTHER" FUEL GROUP	PORTION GUIDELINES FOR WEIGHT LOSS
ALL SUGARS • ALL cakes, cookies, frozen desserts, pies, including FAT-FREE VERSIONS • ALL candies, including chocolates • ALL sodas, excluding diet	**Proceed with CAUTION:** ½ baseball amount = 1 serving of sugars, such as cookies, pie, cake, ice cream 1-2 ping pong balls = 1 serving of most candy, chocolates

THE "OTHER" FUEL GROUP	PORTION GUIDELINES FOR WEIGHT LOSS
ALL FATS **SATURATED:** • Bacon (2 slices=1 ping pong ball) • Butter • Cream cheese • Coconut and products made with coconut or palm kernel • Mayonnaise and salad dressings made with mayonnaise	**Proceed with CAUTION:** (Fats are divided into two types: saturated and unsaturated. You will learn much more about these types in Week 4.) Up to 3 (*women*) or 4 (*men*) ping pong balls daily (1 ping pong ball=1 tablespoon).

• Sausage (1 patty/link = 1 ping pong ball) • Sour cream **UNSATURATED (preferred)*:** • ALL oils and oil-based dressings, except coconut and palm kernel oil • Avocados • Some margarines • Olives, black and green	NOTE: If reduced-fat product is used, you may double the serving size.
SPECIAL FATS: • ALL FRIED foods • ALL pastries (like doughnuts) • HIGH-FAT breads (like biscuits and croissants) • ALL cream-based casseroles	**LIMIT to NO MORE THAN 2** of these "special fats" per week. 1 serving = about 1 baseball (*women*) and 1 ½ baseballs (*men*)
THE "OTHER" FUEL GROUP	**PORTION GUIDELINES FOR WEIGHT LOSS**
ALL ALCOHOL: • Beer (12 ounces) • Light Beer (serving varies) • Liquor (1 ½ ounces) • Wine (5 ounces) Ounces listed indicate amount in one serving.	**Proceed with CAUTION:** Alcohols are concentrated carbohydrate calories that act more like fats after consumed. Count each serving of alcohol as one of your fat servings (**1 serving=1ping pong ball of fat)** *Moderation is considered:* 0 – 1 serving/day (*women*) 0 – 2 servings/day (*men*)

A CLOSER LOOK AT SUGARS

Let's talk about how to handle each of these "Other" fuels: sugars, fats, alcohol, separately, starting with **SUGARS**. In Week 4, you will learn a lot more about the two types of carbohydrates, grains (or starches) and sugars, and how the body uses them differently. In the meantime, you can proceed with caution and deal with your "sweet tooth" in several ways:

1) *You can choose dessert in place of your roll or serving of other starch/grain),* but be aware that you give up vitamins, minerals, fiber, and the type of carbohydrate energy that is "long lasting."

2) *You can choose to have dessert as an **extra** to your meal,* but be aware that it IS extra calories. Try to eat it within 30 minutes of your meal, to take advantage of the other fuel groups present. The fiber and protein from foods like meat and vegetables will slow down your body's response to the quick rush from sugar.

Regardless, keep a close eye on your hunger and fullness level. If you choose option #1, you will hopefully be quite full from the other fuels at your meal and consume only a small amount of dessert as a result. You CAN eat AGAIN, remember! If you choose option #2, remember that a large portion of dessert after a balanced meal can send the extra fuel spilling out of your gas tank into your fat stores. So why not savor the best two bites of any dessert-the first, and *last*, bite! Save the rest for later when your body is more capable of burning it. And who knows? You might even decide that those two bites satisfy your need for sweets, and your desire for the same dessert is gone by the time your next "fuel" break rolls around!

A CLOSER LOOK AT FATS

Now let's look at **FATS**, especially how to handle those special fats. Limit your added fats, like salad dressings and mayonnaise, to an *average* of no more than 3 (women) or 4 (men) ping pong ball amounts daily. On certain days, you may find that you have only one or two. Other days, you may discover that you had five or six before you realized it! But you averaged only three ping pong balls per day, so the amount of fat used will balance out in the end. Special fats, like creamy casseroles, cheesy combination-style foods such as enchiladas, or fried foods, are best limited to no more than two servings per week regardless whether you are male or female. Use your baseball guideline to keep the portion controlled. For example, are you offered a creamy chicken casserole with rice and vegetables at a potluck style event? Or maybe an enchilada covered in cheese sauce at the local Mexican restaurant? The amount of one baseball for women and around one and a half baseballs for men would be your limit for these special fat choices, and then fill up the rest of your plate with extra vegetables or fruits. What about French fries? Keep it to one baseball portion, which translates to a *small* order at most fast food places. Calories, and saturated fats, in commercial French fries add up fast!

A CLOSER LOOK AT ALCOHOL

Finally, take a look at **ALCOHOL**. Are you surprised that alcohol, made from grain itself, counts as a fat serving? Yes, it is a carbohydrate, although it has 7 calories per gram compared to sugar's 4 calories per gram. But, alcohol is broken down and stored in the body much more like a fat than a carbohydrate. Therefore a serving of alcohol, beer, wine, or liquor counts as one of your ping pong balls of added fat. So if you choose to have a glass of wine with dinner, that would be an ideal time to choose NOT to add the ping pong ball amount of butter on your whole grain roll! Since alcohol lowers your ability to resist overeating and stimulates your appetite, be cautious and consume a full glass of water between every serving of alcohol, just to stay on the safe side and keep you fuller in the process! The American Heart Association (AHA) considers a moderate intake of alcohol to be up to one serving daily for females and up to two servings daily for males. If you do not drink at all, the AHA does not encourage you to start.

These "Other" fuel group foods complement your meals or snacks and do not have to be avoided. They are certainly made to enjoy and enhance your foods...but the key is what you do **MORE OFTEN**

THAN NOT. Take a minute to notice how you feel and how your body responds to sugars, fats, or alcohol. Does the energy last? Does it increase your desire for even more food? Does it leave you feeling "heavy" and bloated, and just "over the top"? Was it worth it?

Sometimes, a dessert or a high-fat appetizer might be worth it, because it is a special occasion or just *because*. But it is important to know that your fuel choice was probably made because of the emotional benefits and not your body's actual physical hunger or need for sugar or fats. It may be temporarily worth the emotional effects, but often it may not be worth the longer lasting physical effects, such as the drop in energy, increase in cravings or the extra calories that have nowhere to go but storage.

When you know how to tell the difference between an emotional need and a physical need for a certain food, like that favorite dessert, you keep control of the direction your metabolism is heading. You can enjoy the side trip without the guilt that can keep you sidetracked. The difference in using these foods to complement instead of using these foods to fuel is what makes the difference in your metabolism. In other words, your goal is to choose healthy fuel *more often than not*. Keep an eye on your fuel gauge and your hunger and fullness levels. Soon you will become more in tune with your body and more aware of your reasons *for* your fuel choices and your reactions *to* your fuel choices.

Feeling overwhelmed? How will you remember to balance everything? Anything worthwhile takes an investment in time and energy. Don't try to "get it right" immediately! Here's what you need to do:

A)   **Simply EAT**
B)   **RECORD what you eat**
C)   **CHECK how you did**

You can choose to record your meals or snacks at the end of the day, but you might want to make a quick note on a piece of paper right after you eat and transfer it to your journal later. Regardless, at the end of the day, take a few minutes to check how you did. Did you eat a meal or snack every 4 hours? Did you have 3 to 4 fuel groups per meal? One to 2 per snack? You're making progress! Now, look at your portions. Your plate can be divided into 1/3 protein, 1/3 grain or starch, and the remaining 1/3 full of vegetables and fruit. Check it out-how many baseballs of grain or starch did you eat at a meal? Did you limit the protein at lunch and dinner to the size of your palm? Up to 3 (women) or 4 (men) ping pong balls of added fats daily? Do you see any place you could make changes? More fruit at breakfast? More vegetables at dinner? More turkey on your sandwich at lunch? Less grains everywhere? Simply *learn* and grow closer to your goal of wellness for a lifetime with every step!

Your **FOOD CHALLENGE** for Week 2: **Eat 3 to 4 fuel groups at meals, and 1 to 2 fuel groups at snacks**, using the portion guidelines. Record what you eat in your Maintenance Log.

"Rev It Up! has given me the food groups to choose from, and I was taught how to measure my food by sight without having to weigh or measure anything. It is a great program!"   Michelle

---

WARNING!

Please attempt to build your meals and snacks on your own. Remember, OWNERSHIP is important! But if you need to look at more examples, see the Appendix. A sample day, using grain choices for energy, is provided. For those who avoid grains from either misplaced fear of weight gain or misinformation, a sample day using only vegetable and fruit choices for energy is also included. The Rev It Up! guidelines are flexible and allow you the freedom to choose your own energy and protein sources depending on your preferences. Hopefully, this program will help clear any misconceptions about all the fuel groups over time.

Chapter 7

Headlights on Fluid:
Fill Up Your Water Tank

The key is turned in the ignition, you've been checking your water level, and now you are ready to move your car out of the garage. But if you took the challenge to double the amount of water you drink, up to 8 cups (64 ounces total) of water every day, you may be feeling that the only location you want to move is to the nearest restroom! Yes, you are probably making more frequent side trips to the restroom, but this side effect will not last long!

Your body will adjust to drinking more water by the end of the next few weeks, if not by the end of this week. Your trips to the restroom will begin to subside to once every 2 hours or less. When you get to the finish line of Rev It Up!, 8 cups of water will be your new daily standard!

If you have found yourself behind the challenge at the end of the day, you may have tried to "catch up" by drinking extra in the evening. This is not an effective strategy since you will find that your side trips to the restroom are interfering with a good night's sleep. Recommit yourself to the strategies from Chapter 4 and try to drink water throughout the daytime to avoid nighttime interference.

Just don't give up. Remind yourself that your body is mostly water, and almost everything that happens in your body, including metabolism, depends on a constant supply of adequate water. Water is important for your health and a healthy metabolism.

If this is the first time that you have tried to drink 8 cups of water daily, you may not want to hear that certain circumstances can increase the amount your body needs. You lose water through daily breathing and sweating, so any situation that makes you breathe faster and sweat heavier causes more water loss. Moving your body for exercise is certainly one of those situations! So it makes sense that your need for fluids is even greater when exercise is part of your lifestyle.

You have two choices. If you don't exercise, then your water needs will not increase. But you've learned that exercise gives a boost to your metabolism, so avoiding exercise is really not an option, right? So your other choice is to drink extra when you do exercise!

Do you remember that one of the key functions of water is to act like a radiator to cool your body off when your temperature begins to rise during exercise? What you may not realize is that you sweat about 2 to 4 cups of water for each hour of exercise. This is in addition to the normal amount of water you lose in an hour just from breathing and regular perspiration. If you do not replace this water, your body is not only unable to cool down appropriately but also risks dehydration.

Even mild dehydration can affect your energy level and lead to headaches, dizziness, cramps, even shortness of breath if allowed to continue. Making sure you drink extra water before, during, and after exercise is important to your health as well as your energy and performance. So here's how to fill your fluid level for exercise:

1.   Maintain your "daily 8" cups of water.
2.   Drink an extra ½ cup of water about 30 minutes BEFORE exercise.
3.   Drink an extra ½ cup of water DURING exercise.
4.   Drink an extra cup of water within 30 minutes AFTER exercise.

This equals about 2 cups of extra water on the days you exercise. If you are exercising outside in the heat, you may want to increase even more. Don't wait until you are thirsty to decide to drink. Thirst can be suppressed by exercise or just by habit! Drink enough to satisfy your thirst, and then a little more! You'll keep the radiator cool and your car (or body) performing at its best with just a little extra effort. It's worth it!

Your **FLUID CHALLENGE** for Week 2: **Drink EXTRA for exercise**. Check off the daily 8 cups you now drink and any extra cups for exercise at the top of the page of your Maintenance Log.

Chapter 8

Headlights on Fitness:
Check Your Gas Mileage

What kind of gas mileage are you getting with each mile traveled? Knowing the mileage that you can cover on each tank of gas may not be necessary for actually driving your car, but it is very helpful information.   The efficiency of your gas mileage goes a long way in planning where and when you stop for fuel. And it works in similar ways for your body, too. In other words, are you working hard enough when you exercise to get the most mileage out of your fuel?

If you are new to exercise, or you just started exercising again, you may not feel that you are ready to talk about *working hard enough*. Just getting to the gym, or even putting on your walking shoes, takes planning and effort!   Certainly committing to and beginning an exercise routine is a big step towards improving your fitness for a lifetime. But what if you are not new to exercise? What if you have been exercising for a long time but just don't see the results you thought you would? You faithfully walk on the treadmill or attend that same aerobics class, but you feel "stuck". You can remember feeling stronger the first few months, but now you see little change in your body. Is the effort worth it?

Maybe the problem is not in the effort to get to the gym but in your heart's effort during the time your body is exercising. Is your "gas mileage" efficient-in other words, is your heart really working hard enough to gradually but continually improve your fitness, but not too fast to be dangerous?

The best way to check your gas mileage (quality of performance) is to know your target heart rate range and monitor your workout's intensity. What is a target heart rate? It is the lowest and highest number of heartbeats per minute required to keep you in the aerobic (or oxygen burning) zone, which you learned about in Week 1. You can calculate your target heart rate range and then simply check your pulse during your exercise, or purchase and use a heart rate monitor, which reads your heart rate for you.

A recent study (University of Florida) used heart rate monitors to measure the intensity of the workouts of new exercisers. Although almost 50% rated their work level as moderate, their heart rate monitors showed that *only 15% were right!* Knowing your heart rate takes out the guesswork! Before you calculate your target heart rate, look at the following:

RESTING HEART RATE (RHR):

This is the number of heartbeats per minute when your body is at complete rest. Your heart itself is a muscle, and regular exercise makes stronger muscles. So it makes sense that regular exercise can decrease your resting heart rate since the stronger heart muscle does not have to work as hard to pump the same amount of blood.

Want to calculate your own resting heart rate?
Before you get out of bed in the morning, first thing after waking up when you are lying still and breathing quietly, find your pulse rate and count for 60 seconds. Repeat this for 2 more days and then average the results.

MAXIMUM HEART RATE (MHR):

This is the highest number of heartbeats per minute that your body can give. It can actually be tested only under medical supervision, or you can estimate the number with a simple formula using your age.

Want to calculate your own maximum heart rate?
Pick a formula below (male or female!), insert your age in the blank, and subtract from the first number. The result is your MHR.

(Male) $220 - ($ _____ $) =$ _____MHR
(Female) $226 - ($ _____ $) =$ _____MHR

TARGET HEART RATE RANGE (THR):

Again, this is your aerobic heart rate range-the minimum and maximum number of heartbeats per minute required to get the most out of your exercise time. Remember, aerobic means "using lots of oxygen". The lower end is about 65% of your maximum heart rate, and the upper end is about 85% of your maximum heart rate. Beyond 85%, you move into the "anaerobic" range, where your breaths become shorter and quicker and less oxygen is used as the intensity of the work increases. You can train for brief periods of time in this zone, but the majority of your exercise needs to be between 65 – 85% of your maximum heart rate.

Ready to calculate your own target heart rate?

Multiply your MHR by 0.65 and then by 0.85 to figure out your lowest and highest intensity heart rate range in your target zone:

(MHR _____)x .65 = _____ (lowest intensity THR)

(MHR _____)x .85 = _____ (highest intensity THR)

Divide the lowest and highest intensity THR numbers by 6 to determine what a 10-second heart rate count would be for you (that is an easier number to count when doing aerobic activity):

(Lowest intensity THR ____)÷6 = _____ (lowest 10 sec count)

(Highest intensity THR ____)÷6 = _____ (highest 10 sec count)

NOTE: The formula above is well accepted and designed for average adults who are sedentary or infrequent exercisers. A formula incorporating resting heart rate, which is more individualized and accurate for someone who exercises consistently, will be discussed in Week 6.

Now you can find your pulse on the inside of your wrist and count the number of beats for 10 seconds any time during exercise to know if you are working hard enough but not too hard! The best times to check your heart rate are (1) right after your warm-up to make sure you have entered the aerobic zone, (2) at least once during your exercise, and (3) immediately following exercise. You may want to check your heart rate one final time after the cool-down to make sure your heart rate is back to normal. The amount of time it takes for your heart rate to recover back to your pre-exercise rate is a great indicator of your fitness level. The quicker you recover, the better trained you are and/or the better rested you are. So keep an eye on how fast your heart rate recovers after working out to track improvements in your fitness level as the weeks go by.

Your heart rate range is the best way to check your level of work, but many things can lower or raise your heartbeat outside of exercise alone. Be aware that medications, like over-the-counter medicines for colds or allergies, can raise your resting heart rate. If your resting heart rate is falsely high, your target heart rate range will be affected as well.

Other things that raise or lower your heart rate include, but are not limited to: 1) caffeine from a morning coffee break, 2) outside temperatures--a hot day will increase your heart rate and a cold day will lower it, 3) illness--usually increases your heart rate, 4) use of your upper body during exercise--adding arm or upper body movements will increase your heart rate, and 5) lack of sleep, which can increase your heart rate range depending on how your energy level affects your workout. So use your target heart rate numbers as a guideline only! Pay attention to how your body feels. Always slow down or stop if you feel short of breath, dizzy, or faint.

Another way to pay attention to your target heart rate range is called "perceived exertion." Perceived exertion is simply how intense you perceive the activity to be based on how you feel. The following table will help you monitor your intensity if you don't use a heart rate monitor or the pulse counting method above. Heart rate monitors are relatively inexpensive when you count how many times you will use them but this table works just fine, too.

Exercise Intensity Scale

% of THR	How This Level Feels
Up to 65%	"I'm not even working; I'm very comfortable."
65 – 70%	"My heart's beating faster but I could do this a long time. I can even talk to my neighbor at this pace."
70 – 80%	"My heart and body are working hard. Small talk is all I can do now."
80 – 85%	"Okay, this is intense! Yes/No questions only, please!"
85 – 92%	"I can't talk now!"
Above 92%	"Don't even go there!"

Your **FITNESS CHALLENGE** for Week 2: **Check your heart rate once before, during and after exercise** on at least 2 of the 4 days. Record these numbers in your Maintenance Log. Adjust how hard you are working, depending on whether your heart rate is too low or too high.

A Look in the Rearview Mirror

Week 2: Move Your Car Out of the Garage!

Foundation: Eat breakfast within 1 to 1 ½ hours after rising, and do not wait longer than 4 hours between each meal or snack.

Food: Eat 3 to 4 fuel groups at meals, and 1 to 2 fuel groups at snacks.

Fluid: Drink extra for exercise.

Fitness: Check your heart rate (or perceived exertion) once before, during, and after exercise on at least two days

Now, record any changes you notice this week:

Date	Thoughts, Feelings, Body Changes?

Week 3:

Get in Gear

"I feel I have learned to take better care of my body, so my body will take better care of me." T. T.

Chapter 9

Headlights on Foundation:
Follow the Speed Limits

As you continue to work on your meal alignment from Week 2, turn your headlights towards those "have to have them but they can be so annoying" SPEED LIMIT signs. On a busy street, a speed limit provides guidelines for how quickly you travel in order to control the traffic and maintain safety. A speed limit helps protect you from losing control of the car, which can result in an accident or collision. Likewise, during a busy day, a speed limit for meals and snacks provides guidelines for how quickly *or slowly* you eat in order to control your body's response to the fuel and maintain safety from a collision with your metabolism!

Did you know that it requires about 20 minutes before your stomach can communicate with your brain that it has received fuel from food and is satisfied? If you ignore the *speed limit*, you risk losing control of your body's ability to tell you when you are full. If you are not aware that your tank is full, you will probably continue to eat, right? But more fuel (or calories) than your body needs leads to more fuel storage than your body may want! Fuel is stored in your blood or muscles for more immediate, daily needs OR as body fat for long-term surplus. If your fuel tank overflows, and your muscles already have adequate fuel storage, the extra fuel will be made into more body fat. Although your body is being quite efficient when it adds more long-term storage, you may not be as appreciative of the long-term results.

Watching the speed limit or *slowing down* the meal and snack time so that your stomach has time to communicate with your brain that you are full can help prevent, or at least slow down, storage of extra body fat. When you are aware that you are full and satisfied with your meal or snack, you will stop eating before your body has to figure out what to do with the extra fuel it did not need in the first place.

So what are the minimum speed limits for completing a meal or snack?

TWENTY (20) minutes a meal!
….and TEN (10) minutes a snack!

You may be thinking, "Hey, I can finish a meal in 8 minutes flat, and a snack in seconds! To take 20 minutes for a meal and 10 for a snack – I just don't know if I can do that!" You're not alone. Most of us eat too fast, but slowing down can help you eat more realistic portions while enhancing the amount of enjoyment your food gives.

Do you have to literally eat for 20 minutes at mealtime? No, but commit to allowing a full 20 minutes for the meal "experience." Remain at the table, enjoy the company or the solitude, a chance to take a break from the speedway. Think about what foods you just enjoyed, and how they make you feel. Energized? Relaxed? Make a commitment to *not* return to the kitchen for a second serving until you have waited the full 20 minutes and re-checked how hungry you are then. By that point, your brain and stomach will have had time to communicate, and you may be surprised at their responses! The second serving does not look or sound as good as it did before, because you just aren't hungry anymore. Repeat those now-famous words-**"I CAN EAT AGAIN!"** Feel confident that your efforts to follow the speed limits helped you avoid a ticket for a metabolism disaster-eating too much when you are not really hungry. Way to go!

Your **FOUNDATION CHALLENGE** this week: Glance at the clock or your watch when you begin a meal or snack, and challenge yourself to make your eating experience last according to the speed limit sign: **20 minutes to enjoy a meal and 10 minutes to enjoy a snack**. The key is to slow down and let your stomach communicate to your brain that it is satisfied *before* you look for more fuel!

Chapter 10

Headlights on Food:
Paint Your Portions

You have taken a challenge to follow the speed limits. During that time, why don't you sit back a minute and check out your paint job? How "colorful" are your snacks and meals? Why is color important, anyway?

Do you realize that your grocery store, your pantry, and your plate can contain powerful defenses against disease? These defenses rest quietly and patiently in the produce section of the grocery store, but may never make it to your home, and, even more so, on your plate. These powerful, but often overlooked, superstars are vegetables and fruits-the COLOR in your snacks and meals!

The average American eats only 1 ½ servings of fruits or vegetables daily. Think back to your day: How many fruits or vegetables have you had today? Research has shown, over and over, that people who eat more fruits and vegetables, about five or more daily, have half the risk of cancer then those who eat less than 2 servings daily.

Fruits and vegetables, two of your energy fuel groups, continue to amaze scientists because of the depth of benefits they provide, many of which are still not fully understood. Why is everyone so amazed? First of all, these colorful foods provide fiber, which maintains a healthy intestinal track, helps lower blood cholesterol, and may play a significant role in preventing certain cancers. Secondly, these same unsuspecting foods contain a treasure of vitamins and minerals that are the *spark plugs* for your body. Bananas, citrus fruits, potatoes, and tomatoes all contain potassium, a mineral that regulates every heart beat. Did you know that folic acid, found in orange juice and dark green leafy vegetables, maintains healthy blood cells? And, of course, the famous "antioxidants" beta-carotene and Vitamin C are found in bright orange, yellow, red, and deep green fruits and vegetables, like kiwi, ruby red grapefruits, broccoli, sweet potatoes, and watermelon. Antioxidants help protect your cells from damage, boost your immune system, and reduce the risk of heart disease, cataracts, and some cancers. Just think of them as the superheroes of the body. But there's a catch! It all depends on where you get your antioxidants-from a vitamin and mineral supplement, or from food itself?

For years, every time you picked up a newspaper or turned on the television, another health problem or disease had been successfully attacked by antioxidants. Sales of antioxidant supplements went sky high until April 14, 1994. That's when researchers from Finland and the National Cancer Institute dropped the bomb: Not only did beta carotene supplements fail to reduce the risk of lung cancer, they might even *cause* harm. This shocking news resulted from a study of 29,000 Finnish male smokers, who were randomly chosen to be in one of four groups taking one of the following: a placebo, 33,000 IU of beta carotene supplement, 50 IU of Vitamin E supplement, or beta carotene and Vitamin E combination supplement. After 5 to 8 years, those taking the beta carotene had an 18 percent higher occurrence of lung cancer. What happened? The earlier studies that showed lower cancer rates among people who ate fruits and vegetables assumed that it was the beta carotene present in these foods that was the key. But these studies failed to realize that maybe it is not the beta carotene, pulled out and put in a supplement, which turned the cancer around. There must be something else in fruits and vegetables that work with the beta carotene to protect the body from cancer.

What do you do now?

First, reconsider taking a separate supplement for antioxidants alone, like beta carotene. Secondly, and most importantly, do not stop eating fresh fruits and vegetables! There is no reason to worry about the beta carotene in foods. People who eat more fruits and veggies, especially those rich in carotenes, have a lower risk of most cancers. So just taking a supplement containing the antioxidants is not the answer. But eating more fruits and vegetables may be!

The key to cancer prevention appears to be hidden in these colorful foods, and scientists are just beginning to discover what it is. The "secret" components are called phytochemicals-or chemicals that

FIGHT ("phyt") the evil diseases lurking to attack. Hundreds of phytochemicals exist now and continue to be discovered. These powerful chemicals act like antioxidants and slow down growth in the size of tumors and number of cancer cells. Some of the foods that have high numbers of phytochemicals are the same foods that provide you with vitamins, minerals, and fiber. Broccoli, cauliflower, oranges, grapefruits, blueberries, red onions, cherries and red peppers are just a few great sources.

Look at your next meal or snack and ask yourself, "Is it mostly brown? White? Somewhere in-between?" Even a "healthy" meal like a turkey sandwich on wheat, with pretzels, is brown and colorless, lacking the balance of fruits and vegetables that not only add color but also add fiber, vitamins, minerals, and phytochemicals for fewer calories overall. "Painting" your sandwich with green leafy lettuce and a sliced tomato, and substituting crunchy green snap peas or baby carrots for the pretzels, brightens up your plate and your health!

Try one of the following tips to begin "painting your portions":

1.   Choose a different color to concentrate on each day. For instance, Monday can be RED, and even though you are not limited to just RED colors, you can have fun looking for ways to eat more red: strawberries, raspberries, red grapes, red apples, watermelon, cherries, tomatoes, red peppers, red onions, beets. You get the picture-PAINT IT RED!

2.   Keep convenient packages of vegetables and fruits available at all times- small snack size bags of raw snow peas or carrot sticks for munching, fresh fruit cups from the grocery store for snacking, cherry tomatoes to toss on your salad, ready-to-eat salad greens to stuff in your sandwiches.

3.   Frozen fruits and vegetables always provide a quick back-up, especially for someone on the go who does not cook often.

4.   Freeze chunks of banana or washed grapes, and enjoy as a snack or "dessert." The ice cream-like texture and temperature is a refreshing change, especially in the summertime.

5.   Experiment with different cooking techniques. Instead of simply steaming broccoli, try roasting it in a little olive oil, or shredding it for salads.

6.   Try a new vegetable or fruit that you have never tried before, like star fruit, or kale.

7.   Keep dried fruit, like raisins, dried raspberries or dried apricots, in your car for a quick snack when you are on the road. Avoid the high-sugar types of dried fruits, like banana slices, papaya or pineapple.

Your **FOOD CHALLENGE** for Week 3: **Paint your portions by adding five or more colors every day** in any combination of fruits and vegetables. 100% fruit juice can count, but limit it to 1 serving (4 to 6 ounces) per day. And don't cheat yourself-a large entrée-size salad can certainly count for at least 3 servings of color. So this challenge may not be as difficult as you think. Just keep your eyes open for reds, oranges, yellows, purples, blues, greens, and anything in-between! Highlight or circle the daily "colors" consumed in your Maintenance Log.

What About Vitamin and Mineral Supplements?

Ideally, if you eat balanced meals that include fruits, vegetables, whole grains, lean meats, and low fat dairy products, you do not need to take an additional supplement. But realistically? Most people probably don't. As you learn the Rev It Up! principles, you will begin eating more balanced, but in the meantime, consider taking a multivitamin/mineral supplement that provides 100% of the recommended daily allowances and has the USP mark on the label. And women, please take a calcium supplement with Vitamin D daily if you do not consume 3 dairy servings or high-calcium foods daily.

Chapter 11

Headlights on Fluid: Match Up!

You began Week 1 by checking your water level, and you met the challenge to drink 8 cups of water daily. Week 2 continued the challenge by adding extra water for exercise. How are you doing so far? Are you ready for challenge #3? At this point, trying to meet your water challenge may have naturally decreased the amount of any other beverage consumed. In that case, the challenge this week may be easy. So what's your challenge now?

MATCH UP for QUALITY!

Much debate surrounds the question, "Which fluids count?" According to the Dietary Reference Intakes released in February 2004 by the Food and Nutrition Board, any fluid that hydrates "counts" towards your daily fluid needs. Does current research back the long thought principle that coffee dehydrates? Surprisingly, no it doesn't. What about the safety of diet drinks? If the Food and Drug Administration (FDA) approves the safety, can you consume all of your daily fluids from this kind of fluid? Current research does not negate the hydrating effects of any beverage containing coffee or artificial sweeteners.   Therefore, if you are to meet the Dietary Reference Intake guidelines, all of these fluids can count.

But if you want to take the Rev It Up! challenge to match up for quality, you will need to take a second, closer look. If essentially all fluids can count towards your daily needs, it begs the question, "But is that fluid the best choice for my body?" Just because it counts doesn't mean it is the ideal. Rev It Up is all about quality-quality in your fuel choices and quality in your fluid choices. Fluids with caffeine and beverages with artificial sweeteners, even an occasional alcoholic beverage, have a place in anyone's daily fuel plan, but these beverages need to be consumed in moderation if you want to give your body the best-quality fluid with which to run its engine!

Your Fluid Challenge for this week? In addition to your daily 8, match any amount of these other beverages you consume (caffeine, artificially sweetened, or alcoholic) with equal amounts of additional "match-up fluids". Don't worry-you can count fluids like tomato juice, vegetable juice, and low-fat milk, too. For example, if you have a cup of coffee in the morning, simply match this by filling up your cup with an equal amount of water to drink. Or, if you already consume low-fat milk with breakfast in addition to your coffee, then you have matched up your fluids already! (NOTE: You do not have to match up plain decaffeinated coffee or tea if no more than 1 tsp of added sugar, sugar substitute, and/or creamer is included.)

Now it's time to turn your headlights to focus on more detailed information about caffeinated, artificially sweetened, and alcoholic beverages:

CAFFEINE DRINKS:

Many studies over the years list caffeine as a potential diuretic, which works to release stored water from your cells. However, newer studies have indicated that caffeine may or may not act as a diuretic; that does not seem to translate into actual dehydration for the body. Caffeine may not act as a dehydrator even if it does act as a diuretic in your body. But are caffeine-containing fluids the best choice you can make? Can you meet all of your fluid needs drinking coffee or other caffeine drinks? What amount is considered "moderate" for caffeine intake? Rev It Up! is all about taking your health to the next level of wellness. What you do "more often than not" is what makes a difference. Moderation is the key!

So what is considered moderation for caffeine intake? About 300 milligrams (mg) or less, no more than two or three caffeine drinks daily. If you drink more than 300 mg, you may want to consider reducing the total amount you consume. *A note about soft drinks: As a general rule of thumb, the darker the color of the soft drink, the more caffeine it has. But, as you know by now, there is ALWAYS an exception! Root beer has no caffeine, but popular yellow- and orange-colored sodas may have equal or more caffeine than a dark colored cola!*

Check out the table that follows to view the top caffeine culprits and the # of milligrams per serving:

TYPE OF BEVERAGE	MILLIGRAMS OF CAFFEINE
COFFEE:	
Brewed, 8 ounces (1 cup)	50-150 mg (avg of 100 mg)
Instant, 8 ounces	30-120 mg (avg of 75 mg)
Sweetened mix, 8 ounces	40-80 mg (avg of 60 mg)
TEA:	
Brewed, 8 ounces (1 cup)	20-100 mg (avg of 60 mg)
Instant, 8 ounces	30-70 mg (avg of 50 mg)
SOFT DRINKS:	
Mountain Dew, 12 ounces	54 mg
Colas, 12 ounces	36-46 mg (avg of 41 mg)
Diet colas, 12 ounces	35-46 mg (avg of 41 mg)
OTHER:	
Milk chocolate, 1 ounce	6 mg
Semi-sweet chocolate, 1 ounce	14-35 mg
Chocolate milk, 8 ounces	20-25 mg
Excedrin, 1 tablet	75 mg
Cold medicine, 1 dose	30 mg

To help you determine how much caffeine you really drink, complete the table below. First, list the number of cups you drink of each beverage. Second, multiply the number of cups for each beverage by the specific number of milligrams of caffeine for that beverage, and record the total in the last column. **EXAMPLE:** If you drink 3 cups of brewed coffee daily, your total number of milligrams of caffeine from the coffee would be 300 mg (3 x 100 mg per cup = 300 mg). Now it's your turn:

TYPE OF BEVERAGE W/ CAFFEINE	NUMBER OF CUPS	AVERAGE # OF MG OF CAFFEINE	TOTAL # OF MG PER BEVERAGE
Coffee, brewed		100 mg	
Coffee, instant		75 mg	
Coffee, sweetened mix		60 mg	
Tea, brewed		60 mg	

Tea, instant		50 mg	
Mello Yello, Mt. Dew or Sundrop		54 mg	
Diet Mello Yello, Mt. Dew, Sundrop		54 mg	
Soft drink, dark-colored		41 mg	
Diet soft drink, dark-colored		41 mg	

Now, add the total number of milligrams of caffeine per beverage (column #4) to see the "grand total" amount of caffeine you consume daily._____

If you drink more than 300 milligrams of caffeine daily, consider reducing the amount of caffeine by about 25% for the first 3 or 4 days. But reduce your caffeine very gradually! Caffeine is addictive, so your body may experience some withdrawal symptoms, like headaches, shakiness, and irritability, if you reduce it too quickly. If you have ever had a "caffeine headache", you *know* how your body reacts if you drop your caffeine level too fast! Once you have adjusted to the first reduction, decide if you want to continue reducing even more. Whether you decide to stay at a 1 or 2 cup level, or eliminate it altogether, your body wins!

TO SUMMARIZE: For every cup of caffeine-containing fluids you consume, make sure you consume an appropriate "match up" fluid sometime during the day, such as tomato or vegetable juice, low-fat milk or an additional 8-ounce cup of water. And if you regularly consume more than 300 mg of caffeine, consider reducing the overall amount of caffeine you drink every day.

ARTIFICIALLY SWEETENED DRINKS:

Now let's move on to another popular drink: a "diet" or artificially-sweetened beverage, with or without caffeine. According to the Food and Drug Administration (FDA), it is safe and acceptable to consume foods and beverages sweetened with any of the current artificial sweeteners seen in the marketplace: aspartame, saccharin, acesulfame potassium, neotame, sucralose, and stevia. However, the reports on side effects from artificial sweeteners remain somewhat controversial. Some individuals report that artificial sweeteners like aspartame or sucralose not only stimulate their appetite but may also encourage water retention. It is important to pay attention to how your body responds to these drinks and consider the amount you are currently consuming.

Let's check out the daily acceptable amount of aspartame, one of the most popular types of artificial sweetener. FDA has established 25 milligrams per pound of body weight as acceptable. So if you are 150 pounds, that would mean that your acceptable daily limit is 3750 mg/day (150# x 25 mg per #). Want to calculate your acceptable daily limit? Put your current weight in the first blank and multiply by 25 mg:

(_____ #) x 25 mg (per #) = _____ mg per day

Wow! That is a lot, regardless of how much you weigh! How much is in foods? One packet of aspartame contains 35 milligrams (mg). Diet hot cocoa and diet gelatin each contain about 90 mg. And a diet soda, 12 ounces, contains about 170-195 mg (about five packets of aspartame).

It is doubtful that you consume anywhere near the upper limit of FDA's guidelines for a safe daily amount. However, that does not necessarily mean that more is better, either. One or two diet drinks can fit easily in your day, but repeated and excessive use of any artificially sweetened product replaces the opportunity to choose the best quality for your body. The long-term effects of repeated and excessive intake of artificial sweeteners aren't fully understood yet, even if their use is considered safe. Side effects reported over the years since artificial sweeteners were introduced range from an increase in appetite and sugar cravings to headaches and nausea. Because of these side effects, even if limited to a very small group of people, consider diet drinks as one of the beverages on the Match Up list.

TO SUMMARIZE: Try to limit your intake to no more than 2 daily servings of food or drink that contain artificial sweetener, and match up what you consume with an equal amount of other appropriate fluids (tomato or vegetable juice, low-fat milk, or extra water).

ALCOHOLIC DRINKS:

You have discovered that alcohol is a concentrated carbohydrate but is stored in the body much more like fat than sugar once it is consumed. That is why you count a serving of an alcoholic beverage as one of your ping pong balls of fat (See Chapter 6 for a quick review). But regardless of how it is stored in the body, alcohol also needs to be in the "match up" fluid category because it dehydrates. So for every serving of alcohol (12 ounce beer or light beer, 5 ounce glass of wine, or 1 ½ ounce serving of liquor), match up by consuming an extra 8 ounce glass of water. An added benefit? The water between servings will help subdue the effect of alcohol on your appetite and cravings, too.

WHAT ABOUT THOSE NEW
FITNESS AND FLAVORED WATERS?

You may be saying to yourself, "But I just don't like plain water! What about all those cool new specialty waters? Can I drink those instead?" These products deserve a closer look:

Fitness Waters: These waters are typically lightly flavored, sweetened with a blend of natural and artificial sweeteners and include small amounts of vitamins and/or minerals to help replace fluid losses in an active person. It can be a first step, but the use of artificial sweeteners has other considerations (as you know now!).

Vitamin Waters: These waters are usually sweetened with sugars and contain significant amounts of vitamins and herbs. Check the label – some of these contain as much sugar in 8 ounces as a typical can of regular soda! And the use of herbs can be a concern, especially if you are on medications.

Flavored Waters: These waters are usually calorie-free alternatives, flavored entirely with artificial sweeteners. Similar to a diet soda, without the carbonation.

Oxygen Waters: Just plain water "infused with extra oxygen". Some claim they have more than 10 times the oxygen content of regular tap water-and therefore improve energy, athletic performance, recovery time and brain skills. That's quite a promise! But the American Council on Exercise along with the University of Wisconsin at LaCrosse recently tested these claims and found that "oxygenated water is no more beneficial than regular tap water because there is no physiologic mechanism to get that oxygen in the blood stream where it can be used."

Caffeinated Waters: Water that contains as much caffeine as an 8-ounce serving of coffee-and usually free of sugar, calories, preservatives, and carbonation. But do we REALLY need more caffeine choices?

Lots of choices, lots of options. How can you decide? Think Rev It Up! and think fluid quality!

Are you drinking enough quality fluids?

So how do you know if you are drinking enough to meet your fluid needs with the highest quality choices possible? Ask yourself the following questions:

1. *Are you thirsty?* Thirst usually controls how much fluid you drink. But it can also be a delayed response and therefore not as reliable. For example, when you exercise and sweat, you lose lots of water but exercise itself can blunt your thirst trigger for a period of time. And small children as well as older adults have a thirst system that is not as sensitive and often find themselves dehydrated. Don't always wait for thirst alone to tell you that more water is needed!

2. *Is your urine clear?* If you are becoming dehydrated, your urine may be darker because the kidneys end up

concentrating the fluids when less is available. If your body has enough water to go around, urine usually remains clear and diluted. However, there are two exceptions to this rule.

Exception #1: If you are taking a multivitamin supplement and it is providing more of the water-soluble vitamins (the B vitamins, and Vitamin C) than your body needs, your urine will be more yellow or maybe even orange. For example, if you have plenty of Vitamin C in your blood and body tissues, your body will simply release the extra through "water" in your urine. This extra darkens the color of your urine, just like dehydration can.

Exception #2: If you drink a lot of caffeine-containing beverages, your urine can appear clear and diluted. However, the clear color may not be from adequate hydration but from the fact that caffeine dilutes the concentration of the water present.

Can you drink TOO many fluids, especially water?

You've asked if you are drinking too little water. Can you drink too much? Anything can be done in excess. However, water intoxication, drinking way too much water, is rare in the average population. If you have kidney disease or high blood pressure, especially if you are on medications and treatments to control these, your water intake needs to be moderated by your physician.

People who struggle with compulsive addictive behaviors such as an eating disorder can also drink too much if using water to avoid eating foods yet are already at an unhealthy low body weight. Endurance athletes who run for long distances and do not replace the sodium and potassium that is lost in their sweat can be at risk if they drink plain water without adequate electrolytes. So consuming too much water can certainly be harmful, but it is not common. If you are going to the restroom every 2 hours or so, you are drinking enough but not too much. If you are going more frequently than this, you may want to look at the amount of caffeine, for example, and decrease those beverages instead of automatically decreasing your water intake. They are probably more of the culprit than your water intake itself. Remember, your body is good at getting rid of what it does not need, but it cannot get more water unless you give it!

"I never thought I'd be able to give up my Diet Mt. Dew, but now I find myself wanting water instead!"   Jan

Your **FLUID CHALLENGE** for Week 3: Circle each caffeinated, artificially sweetened, or alcoholic beverage you consume daily in your Maintenance Log, and challenge yourself to **match up amounts of these "other" drinks** with one of the higher quality fluids (water, tomato or vegetable juice, or low-fat milk).

Chapter 12

Headlights on Fitness:
Pump for Power

You have been moving your body and working on your aerobic fitness...now you're ready to shift into gear and experience Pump Power!   Aerobic, or cardiovascular, exercise burns more calories and uses more oxygen, but strength training builds the muscles that heat up your body and increases how fast you burn calories at ANY time, even while sitting! Strength training not only increases muscle mass but also increases the muscle's activity level, or the speed at which the body "makes up and breaks down" protein within your muscle tissue. In addition, strength training also strengthens your bones, which helps reduce your risk of developing osteoporosis. That's reason enough!

Do You Have to Bulk Up?

No! And in fact, if you are a woman, your body is not capable of producing the bulk that can result from strength training, or weight lifting, in men. Your body is not designed that way! Regardless of whether you are a man or a woman, you do not need to "bulk up" to start "melting" your metabolism. Even a little more muscle gained means a little more calories burned when resting. And that leads to better control over your weight! So how do you increase the amount of muscle you have? By pumping for power, or engaging in strength training.

How Much Time Do I Need to Spend?

To pump for power, your goal is to lift weights or use strength training machines or natural body weight exercises two days a week. The goal? One to three sets each of eight to ten resistance exercises to build strength and increase muscle mass. Keep in mind you should try to train A) big muscles before small ones and B) core [central trunk or torso] muscles in addition to upper and lower body muscles.

Your stomach (abdomen) and back muscles serve as the body's *stabilizers* and provide *balance* for your entire body. Your abdominal muscles are actually three sheets of muscle fiber that crisscross completely around you like an old-fashioned girdle, holding in organs and helping hold your entire body upright. If you do not have core strength in these sheets of muscles, you increase the chances of injury when you move weights away from your body. Improved abdominal strength can also "translate into better performance from your body during daily activities" according to the American Council on Exercise (ACE) personal trainer manual. And that will improve quality of life.

Regardless of which muscle group you are working, try to work up to 8 to 12 repetitions per set of each exercise, with a goal of using enough weight that can be lifted at least eight but no more than twelve times. How do you do this? Constantly challenge yourself to add a little more weight, or 1 more repetition, every week or two as you train for strength. If you always lift the same amount of weight the same number of times, you will not get stronger after a period of time. When you are able to do the specific exercise more than 12 times, it is time to add more weight to your routine. And to challenge your muscles even more, try a different exercise for the same muscle group every month or two (More information on these concepts coming in Chapter 18).

Do not feel that you have to add more days, however. Your rest days are very important, since strength training actually tears your muscle tissue, and the new strength and tissue gains you are trying to achieve result from the repair of these tissue tears during rest. In fact, it may be harmful to perform strength exercises for the same muscle group on two consecutive days. Rest at least 48 hours before strength training those SAME muscles again!

Do You Burn Calories Even AFTER the Activity?

Your metabolism can stay revved up after you do any kind of exercise, but the actual number of additional calories burned after exercise varies widely. It depends on the type of workout, and how hard and how long you worked. Many studies have shown that strength training may have a longer "after-burn" of calories than aerobic exercise. One reason may be that this type of exercise raises the level of a hormone called epinephrine, which stirs up metabolic rate. Another reason may be that your body uses up more energy to repair the damage done to your muscles by weight lifting. Regardless of why, exercise like strength training is important for a meltdown of your old metabolism and a jumpstart to a newer one!.

Your **FITNESS CHALLENGE** for Week 3: Make an appointment with yourself to go to the gym, or stay at home and use hand held weights or natural body weight and **pump for power (strength train) 2 days a week**. It need not take more than 30 minutes, depending on how many repetitions and sets are done. Your schedule may not permit-and your goals need not include-more than four hours of exercise time per week. No problem! Simply combine your aerobic activity and strength training on two of the four days. For example, spend 20 or so minutes (including a 5-minute warm-up and cool-down) doing your aerobic activity, like walking or running on a treadmill. Then spend the rest of your time, about 30 minutes, strength training. Save 5 minutes afterwards to complete your stretches. And you are done!

To help keep track, record the total amount of time you participate in exercise, specifically in pump power, in your Maintenance Log. Be sure to make a note of any increase in repetitions or weight, as you progress. And watch your metabolism start shifting!

Is Strength Training a New Concept for You?

Many people, especially women, do not feel comfortable with strength training. You may be one of those individuals! Again, think *small* and *practical*. Put a simple, practical pattern into place and as your routine slowly becomes habit, you will find yourself more at ease with the use of weights to build and strengthen your muscles. An "At-Home Strength Training Starter Program" follows to help you get started.

At-Home Strength Training Starter Program

Although many people make the time and effort to do aerobic exercise, strength training can be more intimidating and challenging, especially if you are not familiar with a gym or the use of weight equipment. Because you may not be a member of a fitness center and unfamiliar with strength building exercises, the following program provides an at-home, simple strength training guide to help get you started. This program can also be followed when you are traveling or are limited in space or time.

WHAT YOU NEED:
A set of 3# hand held weights (dumbbells)
A set of 5# hand held weights (dumbbells)
A set of 10# hand held weights (dumbbells)

As you progress, you can increase your weights by holding either both the 3 and 5# weights in each hand for an 8# dumbbell OR both the 5 and 10# weights for a 15# dumbbell. Eventually you may want to invest in additional hand held weights, up to a 20# set.

WHAT TO DO:
1. Perform 1 to 3 sets of each exercise.
2. Complete 8 to 12 repetitions
3. Do each repetition for 6 seconds, 3 seconds up and 3 down
4. Use a weight that can be lifted at least 8 times but no more than 12.
5. REST at least one day in between strength training

WHERE TO BEGIN:
Start with your lower body (hips, legs and butt muscles), follow with your upper body (chest, upper back, and arms) and finish with your "core" muscles (abdominals and lower back). The following exercises are in this order for you already:

SQUATS: Start by holding a 3 to 5# dumbbell in each hand. Stand with feet a little more than shoulder width apart, holding your abdomen tight and keeping your chin and chest lifted, shoulders open (not rounded forward). Lower your body, without lifting your heels, until your thighs are almost parallel to the floor. Remember to keep the weight in your heels (you should be able to wiggle your toes in your shoes). Hold for 3 seconds and then return to your starting position over the next 3 seconds. Remember to keep your hips above your knees and do not arch your back. Beginners may want to try this without weights and place a chair behind them so that they go down with their buttocks and barely touch the chair before returning to the start position. You may also want to grasp a bar placed over your shoulders and behind your head (a broom or mop will do) to keep your chest lifted. Repeat this exercise 8 to 12 times for 1 to 3 sets. As you become stronger, you may increase the amount of weight that you hold in your hands.

PUSH UPS: Start on your hands and knees, with your hands slightly wider than your chest. Keep your lower legs on the floor, but walk your hands slightly forward, keeping your shoulders, hips, and knees in a straight line. Lower your chest over a 3 second count towards the floor, then push back up to your starting position over the next 3 seconds. Repeat this exercise 8 to 12 times for 1 to 3 sets. As you become stronger, you can change your position by keeping your knees on the floor but lifting your lower legs. Push up as before, over a 6 second count. As you get stronger, you can position yourself in the third, or hardest, position, which requires lifting your knees and lower legs, keeping only your hands and balls of your feet connected to the floor. Your hands should be slightly wider than your chest and your feet about shoulder width apart. Repeat the 3 second count as you lower your body towards the floor. Remember to keep those abdominal muscles pulled in. Regardless of the position used, beginning to advanced, keep your back slightly arched, and don't allow your back to drop below your shoulders.

BENT-OVER DUMBBELL ROWS: While standing on the left side of a bench or chair, rest the right leg (the one closest to the bench or chair) by bending at the knee and placing the lower leg on the bench. Slightly flex the opposite left leg at the knee, keep your spine neutral, and bend at your waist to rest your right hand on the bench or chair seat. Hold a 5-10 pound dumbbell in the hand farthest away from the bench. Extend this arm toward the floor, with the palm of the weight-bearing hand facing towards your side. Pull the dumbbell straight up toward your mid-back, keeping elbow close to your side. Pause; return arm to extended position. Repeat this movement 8 to

12 times, alternating arms for a total of 1 to 3 sets. As you become stronger, you can increase the amount of weight you hold in your hand.

BICEP CURLS: Stand with your feet shoulder width apart. Hold 3-5 pound dumbbells in each hand with your palms facing toward your sides. Keep your elbows at your side and curl the dumbbell upwards over 3 seconds, rotating your palms up towards your shoulders. Then lower the dumbbells back to your starting position over the next 3 seconds. Repeat this exercise 8 to 12 times for 1 to 3 sets. As you become stronger, increase your weights.

TRICEP KICK-BACKS: Stand with your feet shoulder width apart. Hold 3-5 pound dumbbells in both hands with elbows at your side and your palms facing each other. Bend your arms at the elbow so that your forearms are parallel to the floor. With your elbows at your sides, extend or "kick back" your arms over 3 seconds, turning your palms upwards towards the ceiling to isolate the triceps muscles. Slowly return to your bent-arm starting position over the next 3 seconds. Repeat this exercise 8 to 12 times for 1 to 3 sets. As you become stronger, increase your weights. (You may also wish to do single arm kickbacks).

ABDOMINAL CRUNCHES: Lie down on your back with your knees bent and feet flat on the floor. Cross your arms in front of your chest (easier) or place your hands behind your head (harder), and tighten your abdominal muscles. Raise your shoulders off the ground over a 3 second period, keeping the small of your back on the floor at all times. Keep your neck relaxed, using your arms to support your head and not to lift your upper body. Think about your eyes focusing on the ceiling and imagine a baseball under your chin so that you don't bring your chin into your chest. Slowly lower your shoulders back (but not all the way down) towards the floor over the next 3 seconds. Repeat this exercise for 1 to 3 sets at 25 repetitions per set. As you become stronger, you may increase the number of repetitions and/or sets. For variation, as you raise your shoulders off the ground, twist your right shoulder towards the opposite knee to work your oblique (side) abdominal muscles. Alternate by using the left shoulder and twist towards the opposite knee. Repeat 1 to 3 sets of 25 repetitions each.

<u>LOW BACK:</u> Lying face down with hips pressed into floor and abdominal muscles contracted, lift right arm and left leg. Pause and return to the floor. Repeat on the opposite side. Make the exercise more difficult by lifting your arms and legs at the same time, and hold for longer counts during each contraction. Be careful not to over extend your arms and legs-this is a small movement. Stop this exercise (as with any exercise) if you feel pain.

A Look in the Rearview Mirror

Week 3: Get In Gear

Foundation: Follow the speed limits: 20 minutes to enjoy the meal experience, 10 minutes to enjoy the snack experience.

Food: Paint your portions by adding five or more colors every day in any combination of fruits and vegetables.

Fluid: Match up caffeinated, artificially sweetened, and alcoholic beverages with an equal amount of one of the "match up" fluids (low-fat milk, tomato or vegetable juice, water).

Fitness: Pump for power (strength training) 2 days/week.

Now, record any changes you notice this week:

Date	Thoughts, Feelings, Body Changes?

Week 4:

Tune Up!

"I can't begin to tell anyone how Rev It Up! has changed my life. It is very easy principles being applied. Today I am 40 pounds lighter, my portion control is much better and I am much more conscious of what I put into my mouth. I knew the basic concepts of losing weight and keeping it off but just the word exercise made my head ache. But now, I went from a waist size of 38 to 32 and pant size from nearly 20 to a 14. If it was not for this program, I would probably still be at that 202 or heavier. My blood pressure has dropped, my cholesterol level is better, and I am much more energetic."   Kathy

Chapter 13

Headlights on Foundation:
Recheck Your Fuel Gauge

By now, you are well on your way to building a new foundation for a revved up metabolism! You have been concentrating on your fuel gauge, or hunger/fullness levels, before and after each meal or snack. You followed this with meal alignment, the "what" and the "when". Next, you began watching your speed limits for your meals and snacks. It's time to see how much progress you have made! Let's look back since you started Rev It Up!, how many changes have you made? Check off any and all of the following:

- Are you eating breakfast every day (or almost every day)?
- Drinking your daily 8 cups of water?
- Doing an aerobic activity regularly?
- Choosing 3 – 4 fuel groups to build a meal, 1 – 2 to build a snack?
- Trying to eat within 4 hours of the previous meal or snack?
- Eating protein at every meal (dairy or animal/plant protein)?
- Limiting your added fats to 3 ping pong balls daily (4 for men)?
- Limiting special fats, like creamy casseroles and fries, to twice weekly?
- Drinking more water when you exercise?
- Pumping for power by strength training twice a week?
- Concentrating on eating five or more "colors", or fruit and vegetable servings?
- Watching your speed limits by slowing down at meal times?

If you said "yes" to at least two of the above, you are making a significant difference in your health already. Now turn your headlights specifically on your fuel gauge, your hunger (H) and fullness (F) cycle, since this is one of the most important signals that your body uses to communicate with your brain. If you have been recording in your Maintenance Log, look over the numbers you wrote in the "H" and "F" columns, and ask yourself the following:

- Do I wake up hungrier now than before I started this program?
- Do I realize that I am hungry before 4 hours pass between my last meal or snack and the next?
- Can I distinguish more of a variation now between my levels of hunger and fullness?
- Do I notice a positive change in my energy level throughout the day?
- Do I notice that my cravings for sugars and fats are more controlled?

If you are able to answer "yes" to any one of these questions, you are seeing proof-positive signs of a metabolism that is turned on, backed out of the garage, and hopefully in 1st or 2nd gear by now. Congratulations!

Your **FOUNDATION CHALLENGE** for Week 4: **Plan a victory lap!** Choose a reward for your hard work-one that doesn't center around food-and celebrate *you* and your success so far. Record all of the changes you have made in the first month's box on the Victory Lap page (Page 249), and make sure you choose a reward for your hard work. And don't forget to actually make the reward happen for you… soon!

Chapter 14

Headlights on Food (Part 1):
Check the Carb Quality

As part of your Week 4 tune up, it's time to turn your headlights on the *quality* of your fuel choices. This chapter concentrates on the quality of your carbohydrate fuel and the following chapter takes a closer look at the quality of your fat fuel. Carbohydrates and fats are getting lots of media attention now and, frankly, the information can be conflicting and confusing. Carbohydrates, the most important fuel source for your body's muscles and brain, have taken on a heavy burden in recent years as the main reason America continues to gain weight. But a low-carbohydrate approach is heavy on protein and often full of fat. Is this the answer to America's obesity problem?

The high-protein diet was actually one of the very first fad diets introduced in America *over 30 years ago*. Can a high-protein, low carbohydrate diet produce weight loss? Sure! But at what cost to you? If body weight is a combination of mostly water, and other vital components like muscle, organs, bone, and, yes, fat, what exactly are you losing when you lose weight? Are the immediate benefits really worth the possible long-term health consequences?

An extreme approach often leads to an extreme backlash. The result of the first round of high-protein diets was the fat-free craze – almost every food from salad dressings to brownies were made into a fat-free version. Was this the answer? Absolutely not! Fat-free usually means extra sugar. Without protein, and fats, the sugar content increases, the satisfaction factor decreases, and subsequently the total amount of calories eaten continue to increase. Americans began eating less fat than they ever have, but gaining weight!

Both the fat-free craze and the high-protein diet are extremes that significantly decrease at least *one entire food group…a big warning flag* itself! And both can neglect vegetables and fruits-the natural powerhouses of nutrition. Fruits and vegetables are low in calories but high in health promoting fiber, vitamins, minerals, water and phytochemicals-the cancer fighters and immune boosters. High protein diets usually eliminate most of these foods because they are carbohydrates-assumed to be the enemy of weight loss. The fat-free craze, high in simple carbohydrates, also limits these simply because it becomes easier to grab fat-free cookies for a snack than a fruit that may have to be washed and peeled first. So America finds itself eating more, and gaining more weight, so it's back to looking for the next quick fix. Let's stop this crazy, unhealthy cycle!

Take a good look at how the body uses fuel. During digestion, carbohydrates are broken down into glucose, the simplest form of energy required by your cells. Glucose is carried in the blood to be used by the brain, nervous system and, subsequently, muscles for energy.

Every muscle contraction requires glucose, and your brain itself can only be fueled by glucose-about 400 calories daily for the brain alone! When carbohydrates break down into glucose, the length of time it takes varies depending on how much fiber, fat and protein is present. For example, your body works a lot harder to break down lentils into glucose than it does to convert simple sugar fuel, like jelly beans, into glucose.

Your body stores glucose in its muscles and liver, and can store up to 2000 calories at any one time. When you eat, you refuel these glucose stores, and your body uses it between meals to keep it functioning properly. If you exercise between meals, your body is really quick to reach for those glucose stores to fuel the activity. Your meal or snack that follows helps replenish the stores again for the next round.

Are you aware that when your body stores glucose in your muscles and liver, your body adds extra water, in a 3:1 ratio, in the storage process? So stored glucose also means extra fluids stored in your muscles and liver. That's good, because your body *is* mostly water (about 65% +), and water is vital to *every* single metabolism process that occurs-from muscle contractions for a bicep curl to burning stored body fat.

So what happens when a person significantly restricts the body's most important fuel source, glucose? For the first 3 days, your body ignores the protein or fat that might have been eaten and looks for whatever stored glucose it can find in the muscles and liver. Guess what happens next? As glucose is released to be used by your brain or a muscle, so is water! In a few days, your glucose energy stores are fairly depleted, and you get on the bathroom scale, and WOW! Weight loss! Really? Actually, mostly *water* loss – not body fat loss. *The average female can lose only about 1 to 1 ½ pounds of body fat per week, and the average male can lose only about 2 to 2 ½ pounds per week.* So any weight loss greater than these amounts within a week's time is not fat. What's left? Water, and muscle, and even bone, over time.

Once your stores of glucose are used up, your body begins trying to adapt to its circumstances in an effort to maintain life. So, it begins forcing itself to use the protein you are eating as fuel from which to make new glucose. It can convert a piece of chicken into glucose if it has to, but at greater effort and less efficiently than it would whole wheat bread. Your body can also just as easily eat its own muscle if fuel is not readily available, and, in fact, it will do so under the strain of a high-protein diet over a period of time. And, yes, fat stores are used, too-but again not as predominately as you'd like to believe.

The process of breaking down protein and fats, the predominant fuels in steak, eggs or cheese, to glucose can lead to a condition called ketoacidosis. Any medical professional will tell you that if a hospital patient went into ketoacidosis, it is considered a state of alert-and a sign of starvation. For example, if a cancer patient tested positive for ketones, a registered dietitian would be called in quickly to help change the food intake level and type to prevent, or stop, this condition. And a high level of ketones is also a warning sign for which a physician looks when testing for diabetes. It is a sign that something in the body is not working as it should, and the body has compromised to survive. Finally, keto**acid**osis, with *acid* being the key word here, increases the body's risk of kidney stones. And, more importantly, ketoacidosis increases the risk of bone loss from the body and decreases the body's ability to recover by forming new bone. How can ketoacidosis, and a high-protein diet, be a good thing now?

Weight loss may continue on a high-protein diet, but realize that it is not just pounds lost from fat. Water loss is a constant problem because protein itself, when it is digested, forms ammonia (a quick chemistry lesson!), ammonia forms urea, and urea will make (you guessed it) urine. So the more protein eaten, the more urine made, and the more water loss. Your poor kidneys are doing double duty! And eventually weight loss may simply continue because you are tired of all that meat and cheese and you just begin eating less of it. Less calories, of course, leads to weight loss, too.

Boredom sets in -- the choices are pretty limited if you avoid most all of the grains, fruits and vegetables suggested. Maybe you break down and have a piece of bread, or a cookie you have been craving. What happens? Well, your body is so thrilled to have the real, usable form of carbohydrate again that it breaks it down readily and returns some glucose to the muscle stores for later use. But remember, glucose is stored with water. Uh oh! What does the scale do? It goes *up* -- seemingly overnight, bread has made you feel "fat" again. No, bread doesn't make you fat like that, but eating a carbohydrate like bread *did* re-hydrate your dried-up muscles-and the scale is weighing in that extra fluid.

But the weight gain itself can be too hard to handle, and the temptation is to avoid all carbohydrates yet again. But avoiding carbohydrates is avoiding your body's most important energy source! The problem is not carbohydrates themselves, but the **quality of the carbohydrate fuel** you choose. Both simple sugars (like jellybeans) and grains or starches (like oatmeal and 100% whole-wheat bread) are carbohydrates that are broken down into glucose; however, how *fast* this process takes place is the key to running out of energy or fueling smart. Smart carbohydrate fuel provides lasting glucose energy that keeps your brain powered up and your muscles fueled.

Carbohydrate like simple sugar found in most candies, cookies and colas breaks down into glucose energy in a very short period of time –less than 30 minutes. Energy is available quickly, but is used up quickly as well. This usually results in a drop in energy level that can not only affect your muscle and brain power but also lead to cravings for another sugar "high" within 1-2 hours. And if your fuel tank itself is pretty full already, all of the quick energy suddenly available has nowhere to turn but to your fat stores to be used later.

On the other hand, high-quality (complex) carbohydrates like whole grains, fresh fruits and vegetables take longer to break down completely into glucose -- since this type of carbohydrate has long chains of starch and more fiber to "work through". Also, add lean protein and a little fat to the same meal, and the process will be slowed down even more, allowing a gradual release of fuel into your body over a longer period of time. So, at a meal that includes 3 to 4 fuel groups, even the simplest carbohydrates like white rice, or a dessert like sherbet, will be released more slowly because of the protein and/or fat present in the other foods at that meal.

Therefore, a balanced meal has a built in buffer - the protein and fat fuel-because they help slow the rate of energy released, used and stored from carbohydrates. But a snack can be more difficult. Will your snack choice give your body low- or high-quality energy? *It all depends on the type of carbohydrate you choose, and if protein and/or fat is included.*

For example, a high-quality snack is an apple, sliced, with natural peanut butter. This combination gives you carbohydrate energy from the fruit, and protein and fat from the peanut butter. If you substitute 100% whole-wheat crackers for the apple slices, you have another good option. But what if you only have saltine or club-type crackers available? These common crackers are white-flour based, processed carbohydrates. The more "processed" a carbohydrate (or in other words, the higher the amount of white flour), the quicker it is broken down into sugars, or glucose-since the manufacturer has done the work for you, and little if any fiber is present. That's where the addition of peanut butter helps! Spreading natural peanut butter on even your "white flour" crackers will slow down the rate in which the crackers are broken down into glucose energy. A slower rate of breakdown means a more stable blood sugar level-avoiding the quick sugar drop that zaps your energy and increases your cravings.

What about graham crackers? They are also broken down fairly quickly, but adding dairy protein like a glass of 1% milk will slow the process down. Likewise, vanilla or lemon flavored yogurt has some added sugar, but the protein from the yogurt itself will help slow down the release of those sugars and encourage a more gradual rise and fall in your energy level. You can use the artificially sweetened yogurts, but you may receive more satisfaction from choosing a yogurt that is not artificially sweetened but still has less sugar than your typical fruit brands. Yogurts that have less sugar include many organic brands, Greek style brands, vanilla or lemon flavored brands and the "fruit on the bottom" brands, since you can control how much sweetened fruit syrup you stir in.

The following list gives you more suggestions for SMART SNACKS for one or two fuel groups. The key is to look for more whole grains and less sweetened, "instant", or "white-flour based" products. Remember: the more processed a carbohydrate, the quicker it is broken down into sugars, or glucose. Pay attention to how your fuel gauge responds. If you are hungry again within an hour, you probably chose a lower-quality fuel that "burned out" quickly, or did not eat any source of protein or fat with it. Learn to snack smart, and choose high-quality fuel that keeps your energy level running smoothly!

Your **FOOD CHALLENGE** (Part 1) for Week 4: Choose a snack combination that will improve the **quality of your carbohydrate fuel**. Continue to record what you eat in your Maintenance Log.

"I love eating the Rev It Up! way. Less amounts of meats, more fruits and vegetables, better choices for grains, more low- fat milk and yogurt. The afternoon snack is wonderful. As long as I eat every 3 to 4 hours, I feel more energized and more in charge of me."   Joyce

Are you still confused on what exactly determines whether a carbohydrate is a "whole grain"? See Question #3 in the "Most Frequently Asked Questions" section of the Appendix.

Smart Snack Suggestions

The following list provides suggestions for smart, high-quality fuel for snacks. The "1 Fuel Group" snacks are more ideal for mid morning-to give you a little boost between breakfast and lunch. The "2 Fuel Group" snacks are ideal for the afternoon, when you have a long stretch between two meals. The added protein or dairy fuel will help the energy from the grain or fruit last longer. Experiment with different choices, and notice how your body responds.

1 Fuel Group Snacks
Any fresh fruit
Dried, unsweetened fruit like raisins or apricots
Carrot sticks or fresh snow peas
Low-fat yogurt or cottage cheese
Mozzarella cheese stick
A "baseball size" amount of pretzels or low fat chips**
Graham crackers, about 1 large rectangle**

2 Fuel Group Snacks
Low-fat yogurt with sliced almonds
Fresh fruit or vegetables with low-fat cottage cheese
Graham crackers and natural peanut butter
Reduced-fat (2%) cheese and whole-wheat crackers
A "mini" whole grain pita pocket and 1 to 2 lean turkey slices
An energy/protein bar (look for about 200 calories, 10+ gms protein)
Apple slices and a mozzarella cheese stick
A banana with natural peanut butter
A mix of whole grain cereal with walnut pieces

**_Proceed with Caution_ with choices like these, since they have a higher percentage of white flour, with added sugar. When eaten alone, expect the energy to last a shorter period of time than fuel choice with more fiber, protein, fat._

***_See Question #13 in the "Most Frequently Asked Questions" section of the Appendix for guidelines on appropriate energy bars._

Chapter 15

Headlights on Food (Part 2):
Check the Fat Quality

Of all the fuel choices you have, which one do you think can have the most powerful long-term impact on your weight and health? If you guessed fats, you're right! Sugars certainly have an impact and can provide a quick rush of calories that overflow the capacity of your gas tank easily; however, fats provide the biggest calorie load in the smallest amount and can add up much quicker than you might realize. It's time to turn on your headlights and take a look at the quantity and quality of the fat fuel in your meals and snacks; in other words, raise that hood and check your oil!

Take a moment to think back to your car. Gas is the fuel for your engine, but it cannot do its work alone. Motor oil works hand in hand to make sure the engine can use the gas efficiently. Oil lubricates the motor, and the quality of the oil used determines how well and how long it will do its job before losing its effectiveness. Oil not only lubricates but also picks up "trash" that is left over from the day's work. This "trash" directly interferes with the oil's ability to lubricate and keep the motor running smoothly for a longer period of time. You do not need nearly as much oil as you do gas, and an oil change will last longer than a tank of gas. But even if the quantity is small, its job is big.

Now compare motor oil to the fats in your foods. In a similar way, the fats that you eat are necessary to lubricate your body's motor and keep it running smoothly. However, different types of fats exist, just like different grades or quality of oils. And some oils are simply full of "trash" that interferes with your body's performance.

Take a moment to check your oil. In other words, let's check the amount and the grade, or *type*, of fat in your daily meals and snacks. Your body does not need nearly as much oil, or fat, compared to foods needed from the five fuel groups, but the right kind of fat is the key to keeping your body performing well!

What does fat in your daily meals and snacks do for your body? Look at this list of functions and see if you are not impressed at the work it can accomplish:

- Fats provide structure for every cell in your body.
- Fats provide linoleic acid, an essential fatty acid that must be obtained from food sources.
- Fats provide transportation for all the fat-soluble vitamins, Vitamin A, D, E, and K. Vitamin A is necessary for healthy skin and eyes, Vitamin D for healthy bones, Vitamin E for a healthy immune system, and Vitamin K for efficient blood clotting. If no fat is available from our foods, these key vitamins do not have any means of transportation to do their job!
- Fats increase satiety from a meal or a snack (in other words, you feel fuller longer), since they contain 9 calories per gram. Proteins and carbohydrates provide only 4 calories per gram. Therefore, adding a small amount of fat can provide a large amount of energy, or calories! This can HELP you if you know it will be at least 4 hours before you are able to eat again.
- Fats, as well as proteins, help stabilize blood sugars, and buffer or slow down the digestion and absorption of carbohydrates. Therefore, the energy you receive from carbohydrates you eat will last longer if that food choice is eaten with a fat and/or a protein.

Pretty amazing, isn't it? You can see the importance of fats, but different grades or types of fats do exist. The two types of fats are **SATURATED** and **UNSATURATED**.

What is the difference in these? A tablespoon of either saturated or unsaturated fat contains the same number of calories. For example, a tablespoon of butter (a saturated fat) equals the same number of calories (about 100!) as a tablespoon of olive oil (an unsaturated fat). But saturated fats actually raise your cholesterol levels and contribute to heart disease, unlike unsaturated fats. Let's take an even closer look at these two types of fats, so you can choose the best grade or quality of oil for your body's motor.

SATURATED FATS

Saturated fat equals <u>animal fat</u>; that's easy to remember. But, there is always an exception to the rule, especially when you are talking about nutrition. (Don't you love it?) Saturated fats from animal foods like meat and cheese are easy to see, but saturated fats from plant foods are not as easy to identify but do exist. These plant food exceptions include coconut (hence, coconut oil), palm kernel oil, vegetable shortening, and margarines that contain *hydrogenated* fat. *Hydrogenated,* or *hydrogenation,* is a key word that indicates saturated fat. Anytime you see this word on a food label, you know that it contains more saturated fat. Soon, all labels will be required to indicate how much saturated fat from hydrogenated ingredients is present. In the meantime, an easy rule-of-thumb that you can use to estimate how much is present is to check out the order of the ingredients on the label itself. The further down the list, generally the less amount of hydrogenated fat used. So what exactly is hydrogenation? It is a chemical process that takes *unsaturated* oil like corn oil and changes it to a semi-solid or solid fat, hence, *saturated.* Another word for this type of fat is *trans fat.*

If hydrogenation makes a fat saturated, and saturated fat is the culprit behind higher cholesterol levels, why is it still used by food manufacturers? It makes a food that normally would not stay fresh be able to last a long time. In other words, it makes that same food shelf stable. Oil can become rancid, changing the smell and taste and quality of the food in which it is used. Hydrogenation prevents this. This is good news to vending machine suppliers! The products in that vending machine will remain fresh for a long time. That is why a food like a quick-stop cream filled sponge cake can sit in that vending machine for months (years?) and taste the same. *If the fat in that food can resist change for that long -- how long can it resist change, or stay solid, in your heart arteries?* Makes you wonder!

Here's a list of saturated fats from animal foods and from plant foods:

SATURATED FATS FROM ANIMAL FOODS	SATURATED FATS FROM PLANT FOODS
Red Meats (Beef, Lamb, Pork)* Dark meat chicken and turkey* Chicken or turkey skin Egg yolks Whole milk and whole-milk cheeses Butter and cream Processed meats, like hot dogs, bacon and sausage *Saturation depends on cut of meat (Ex: prime rib is higher-fat cut; sirloin is lower-fat cut)*	Coconut and coconut oil Palm or palm kernel oil Margarine (with hydrogenated oil as the first or second ingredient)** Vegetable shortening** Products made with hydrogenated oil (such as many vending machine snacks and sweets)** Fried foods cooked in shortening** **These foods contain trans fats, which elevate blood cholesterol.*

Is this list telling you not to ever have these fats? No. Red meats, like beef, lamb and pork, contain high-quality protein, and are rich sources of vitamins and minerals like Vitamin B12, zinc, and iron to name a few. Egg yolks are also great protein sources, full of iron, Vitamin E, and lecithin. The American Heart Association recommends lean red meats up to four times a week, and egg yolks up to 4 times a week. Recent studies have even indicated that egg yolks could be eaten more often than 4 times a week within a balanced diet because the cholesterol in egg yolks did not seem to promote an increase in saturated fats in the study subjects who ate an egg every day. A choice like beef or egg deserves a place on your plate, but the choices to consider most carefully are the saturated fats from certain plant foods and the hydrogenated fats, or trans fats.

To make sure you understand what a trans fat is, let's compare butter and margarine. Butter is from an animal and contains saturated fat. Notice how hard butter is when you remove it from the refrigerator? It takes quite a while to soften! Margarine, on the other hand, is made from oil, an unsaturated fat, which has been made semi-solid or partially hydrogenated through a chemical process. It now remains hard or solid at room temperature from the presence of trans fats, although not quite as hard as butter. Some researchers argue that trans fats can increase the bad cholesterol level in your body as much as a food high in saturated animal fats. But unlike saturated animal fats, trans fats, or hydrogenated oils, can also *decrease* the good cholesterol (explanation of "bad" and "good" cholesterol is coming up!). And we need as much of the "good" cholesterol as possible to protect us against heart disease.

So do you never eat a Twinkie again? Maybe, maybe not – but at least know what you are eating. What if you have to choose between a vending machine snack or going longer than four hours before eating again? Your metabolism will appreciate a snack and having something between meals will help prevent overeating at the next meal. Just try to make the healthiest choice available. Nowadays, many food manufacturing companies are beginning to take notice and produce more products that have less, if any, trans fats. Even vending machines sometimes offer healthier fat alternatives, like low-fat pretzels or heart-healthy nuts. But if a healthier alternative does not exist, an occasional Twinkie is not going to raise your trans fats significantly. If you do not eat from vending machines often and limit processed foods overall, your level of trans fats is probably not a problem.

How do you deal with the other saturated fats, the ones from animal foods? Helpful hints include using lean cuts of red meats, removing the skin of the chicken or turkey, limiting high-fat breakfast meats and substituting lower-fat versions, and moderating the number of egg yolks you have each week. What if you are at your favorite restaurant, and they serve you fresh homemade bread with tiny butter pats (you know, the ones that are shaped like flowers or stamped with the restaurant logo)? It is not the time to ask for a tub of diet margarine, right? You may wish to use that butter on that warm roll. Enjoy the taste and aroma as it melts-but limit to one, and make it last! Sure, you had saturated fat, but within moderation. Not a problem!

UNSATURATED FATS (in other words, SMART FATS!)

On the opposite side, unsaturated fats are usually *liquid* at room temperature and found in plant foods. Unsaturated fats help lower the "bad" cholesterol and reduce your risk of heart disease. Different types exist:

POLYUNSATURATED FATS	MONOUNSATURATED FATS
Corn oil	Canola oil
Safflower oil	Olive oil
Sunflower oil	Peanut oil
Soybean oil	Nuts and seeds, such as the
Fatty fish*, such as the	following: peanuts, almonds,
following:	pecans, walnuts*, pistachios,
Salmon, tuna, herring, sardines,	sesame seeds
mackerel, rainbow trout, halibut,	Nut butters, like peanut butter
Atlantic bluefish, eel, and lake	Avocados
trout	Olives, black and green

Did you know that a fatty fish like salmon, and even walnuts, are high in polyunsaturated fats, specifically omega 3 fatty acids, which protect against heart disease? Omega 3 fatty acids help lower levels of blood fats, reduce blood clotting, help make irregular heart beats less likely, and often increase the production of "good" cholesterol. The American Heart Association has added the recommendation to eat fish, preferably fatty fish, at least twice a week. Concerned about the safety of eating cold-water fish due to information you've heard about mercury levels in the water? The FDA has acknowledged that it is safe to eat fatty fish oils in amounts up to 3 grams of omega 3 fatty acids daily. One serving (3 ½ ounces) of salmon contains about 1 gram of omega 3 fatty acids, so even a daily serving of fish meets the safety guidelines. If you are still uncomfortable, or just don't go for that fishy smell, add walnuts to your meals or snacks daily. They are also a good source of omega 3's.

Okay, you are now aware of the types of fats, saturated (including trans fats), and unsaturated (including fatty fish). Have you noticed the terms "good" cholesterol and "bad" cholesterol have been associated with the different types of fat? Saturated fats increase the bad cholesterol, and trans fats even lower the good cholesterol. What exactly IS cholesterol, and which ones are *good* or *bad*?

CHOLESTEROL

Cholesterol is a waxy-like substance that is found only in animal tissue. Cholesterol is made in the liver by the body, which is the reason why you will only find it in something that has a liver! (A cow, a pig and a chicken all have livers...but a corn stalk does not! Hence, fats in foods from these animals will have cholesterol but corn oil will not.) Cholesterol is very important to your body, because it plays a role in making all of the body's steroids, such as bile salts (which help digest fats), Vitamin D (which helps build strong bones), and your reproductive hormones (you know what those do!). It also gives physical structure to every cell. Your body makes cholesterol in the liver and works to balance the amount it makes with the amount you eat. So, reducing the cholesterol intake from your meals and snacks would probably cause little harm to the body because it can usually make its own. If you eat less cholesterol, your body is designed to make more to meet the demands. Likewise, if you eat more, your body, in most cases, can make less to keep the balance.

The body does have the ability to balance cholesterol, but this ability can be greatly affected by what you eat as well as your family history. The American Heart Association warns that one of the significant risk factors for heart disease is a high level of blood cholesterol. A diet continually high in cholesterol can lead to higher levels of cholesterol in the blood. So it is important to limit the amount of saturated and trans fats in your diet because these fats trigger your body to produce more cholesterol.

Once it's produced, just how does cholesterol get from the liver to the other parts of the body? It takes a ride through the blood stream! This is not as simple as it may sound, because cholesterol and blood are a lot like oil and water...they do not mix well! Your amazing body has a special system of transportation designed to carry cholesterol in the body to where it's needed. It does this in the liver by mixing fats with protein and making different types of "transportation vehicles" called lipoproteins ("lipids", which is another word for fats, plus "protein"). Since blood itself is a protein, it can now mix with fat in the form of a lipoprotein so that cholesterol can be carried throughout your body.

One main type of lipoprotein is the LDL, which stands for low-density lipoprotein. The LDL contains about 60-80% cholesterol, and it really loves to travel and deliver its cholesterol package to the cell walls of the heart arteries. Saturated fats, including trans fats, trigger the production of this type of lipoprotein, the LDLs. Therefore, this lipoprotein is known as the *bad* cholesterol. What can you do to lower the LDLs? *Eat less saturated and trans fat!*

The other main type of lipoprotein is the HDL, which stands for high-density lipoprotein. The HDL contains more protein and less cholesterol (only 20%) than the other lipoproteins. HDLs love to travel to the cell walls of the heart arteries and *remove* the cholesterol deposited by the LDLs. Then the HDLs deliver this cholesterol back to the liver for eventual removal from the body through the intestines. HDLs actually protect against heart disease, so they are known as the *good* cholesterol.

If HDLs are so good for you, what can you eat to make more of them? Sorry, food intake has little effect and no particular food will significantly increase the level of HDLs in your body. But, *exercise will*! That is yet another reason you benefit from the aerobic exercise and strength training you do on a consistent basis.

Who thought checking the oil would be this complicated? Well, let's make it as simple as possible. Here are some common challenges and suggested strategies to improve the grade or quality of oil that goes into your body:

 Continue to moderate or limit the amount of total fat you are eating daily by limiting your fats to no more than 3 "ping pong ball" portions for women, 4 for men, per day. Now, individualize your specific "Check the Oil" challenge and choose your road map:

CHECK THE OIL CHALLENGE #1:
Do you eat a lot of fried foods?
- Eliminate fried foods to no more than twice a week.
- Experiment with oil- and vinegar-based marinades.
- Grill, bake or roast instead of frying.

CHECK THE OIL CHALLENGE #2:

Do you eat a lot of red meat (beef, pork or lamb)?

- Choose lean cuts of red meats, like tenderloin, round or sirloin.
- Limit red meats to no more than four times a week.
- Moderate and balance the number of egg yolks you consume a week, either alone or within a casserole type recipe. You can often substitute egg substitute or egg whites in a recipe without losing the quality or consistency.

CHECK THE OIL CHALLENGE #3:

Do you eat enough omega 3 fatty acids?

- Increase your fish intake on a weekly basis by trying to eat fish, especially cold water fish, twice a week. Add it once a week for the first 2 weeks, and then increase to twice a week. By the end of this program, you will have made fish a regular part of your week!
- Order grilled fish in a restaurant if you do not like to prepare it at home, or take advantage of the precooked fish at your local grocery store.
- Add walnut pieces (at least one ping pong ball amount daily) to your breakfast cereals, home made trail mixes, yogurt or as a salad garnish.

CHECK THE OIL CHALLENGE #4:

Do you eat a lot of higher-fat dairy products?

- Substitute 1% or skim milk products for 2% or whole milk products, like milk, cottage cheese and yogurt.
- Substitute 2% cheeses for whole-milk cheeses, either block, sliced or grated versions. Fat-free cheeses are not necessary. They do not taste or melt like 2% or regular cheeses and can alter a recipe result.

Your **FOOD CHALLENGE (Part 2)** for Week 4: Plan your personal road map by identifying one of the "check the oil" challenges that you face most frequently. Then select one or more steps to concentrate on this week to **improve the quality of your fat fuel.** Record what you eat in your Maintenance Log, noting any improvements in your fat quality as the week progresses.

MY PERSONAL "CHECK THE OIL" CHALLENGE IS:

_____

_____

_____

_____

_____

THE STEP(S) I WILL TAKE TO IMPROVE THE QUALITY OF FAT FUEL ARE:

_____

_____

_____

_____

_____

"Great news! My official weight loss was 17 pounds in 3 months. My overall cholesterol when down from 265 to 202, and my LDL (bad guys!) went down from 169 to 119. My triglycerides went down from 170 to 115. My overall ratio decreased from 4.3 to 3.4-GREAT, huh?" Doris

Chapter 16

Headlights on Fitness:
Check for Safety and F.U.N.

Ready to tune up your fitness program and check for safety? How about checking for F.U.N.? Safety is critical when it comes to your exercise form and body alignment. If the wheels on your car are out of alignment, it can cause extensive (and expensive!) damage. Likewise, if your form is out of alignment, it may cause damage to your body's ligaments and joints. And when it comes to enjoying safe exercise, keeping the F.U.N. is just as important. Let's start with the safety check:

SAFETY CHECK

BREATHING (All exercises):
1. Pay attention to your breathing, and NEVER hold your breath.
2. Stay relaxed and inhale during the down phase of the movement.
3. Stay relaxed and exhale during the up phase or exertion of the movement.

UPPER BODY MOVEMENTS:
1. Avoid swinging your arms-only lift weight that you can take through the movement without momentum.
2. Keep your shoulders and neck relaxed.

LOWER BODY MOVEMENTS:
1. Avoid extending your knees past your toes.
2. Keep your hips above or parallel to your knees.
3. Again, don't swing or use momentum.

ABDOMINAL MOVEMENTS:
1. Avoid lifting your lower back off the floor.
2. Support your neck with your arms without pulling your head and shoulders forward.
3. Keep an imaginary tennis ball under your chin to keep your head in the correct position.

Anything you need to change? Make a mental note or even jot down a reminder on a post-it note and stick it on your treadmill at home, or in your tennis shoes if you work out at a gym or walk around your neighborhood. That way you won't forget when you get ready to exercise again. And make sure you perform a safety check regularly to keep things in line.

The safety check has been covered, so time to move on to the F.U.N. part. Take a few minutes and "play with" your fitness goals right now, and see if you need a F.U.N. strategy to rev things up again!

Make Fitness F.U.N.

F = FLEX your schedule
U = UNDERSTAND your challenges
N = NIX the negatives

F is for FLEX, not your muscles but your schedule! The best way to fit a workout into your life is to schedule it as you would any other appointment. Try blocking off the same times every week, but be realistic. If you know that you are NOT a morning person, there is no need to set that alarm for an early hour and then feel guilty when you hit the snooze button every 5 minutes! Likewise, if you know that the end of the day always includes some kind of interference that prevents you from getting to the gym, schedule your fitness appointment before work or during your lunch hour. And when an emergency happens-at work OR home-and you simply cannot keep your commitment to exercise, handle it as you would any other important appointment. Reschedule, as quickly as possible-and let go of any guilt for doing so when your circumstances have prevented it. If someone you know has to reschedule an appointment with you because of an injury, sickness or a last-minute emergency, you understand and are flexible. Why not offer the same courtesy to yourself?

Flexibility in your schedule is important, but so is flexibility in the *type* of exercise you do! Plan variety into your activities to not only keep the engine warm and your car moving but also simply keep your interest! If you do the same activity over and over, your body becomes very efficient doing the same moves repeatedly and begins burning fewer calories to do the same amount of work. Adding variety each week helps prevent the body from "getting used to it" and maximizes the benefit you receive for your efforts. It also is just a lot more enjoyable!

U is for UNDERSTAND your challenges! Life is full of different seasons - a season for education, a season for work challenges, a season for travel, maybe a season for raising children or taking care of an elderly family member. What specific challenge are you facing in this season of life?

- Young children at home
    - o Understand the limitations on your time.
    - o Swap "babysitting time" with a neighbor to allow you to get to the gym.
    - o Purchase an at-home exercise video, or complete the strength training starter program, when your children are napping or busy.
    - o Find a gym that has reputable childcare and arrange your day to fit activity in during the time it is available.
- Overtime hours at work
    - o Consider exercise a "must" for stress release instead of a way to burn calories, and you might be less likely to miss your exercise appointment.
    - o Split up your exercise time into smaller sessions until your work schedule is relieved.
        - ▪ Walk 20 minutes in the early morning.
        - ▪ Stop by the gym on the way home for a quick 20-minute workout to round out a 40-minute session.
        - ▪ Look for ways to add activity to your every day routines, such as parking your car further away from the office door and taking stairs instead of elevators.

- Compromise by trying to exercise only 1 out of the 5 workdays, but make exercise a priority on both *weekend* days until your work schedule changes.
- Schedule the days you will NOT exercise to release you from guilt about "missing a day"-view it as a day of rest for which you planned.

Whether the challenge lies in the workplace or family commitments, these strategies can help you work around the challenge without neglecting your fitness.

N is for NIX the negatives! The more often you hear something, the more you start believing it. Do you hear yourself say negative statements like "I knew I couldn't stay committed", "I always quit!", "It works for you but it's impossible for me", or "I never can find the time"? You'll eventually start believing it, if you don't already. Try to nix the negatives in its tracks. Be prepared to battle back with positive punches-"I have had a difficult week but I'm starting fresh today", "I will make it work for me, even if I have to make several changes along the way to find the right routine", "I deserve to move and exercise-it makes me feel better!" or "One day at a time is all I have to do!" If you have a choice to be around a friend with a negative attitude or a positive attitude, which one are you most likely to choose? A positive attitude attracts, a negative attitude repels. Begin saying positive statements, and you'll notice how much more you *enjoy* being with yourself!

How about looking for an exercise partner that will keep you accountable while encouraging your progress? As important as finding a good mechanic or body repair shop that you can trust to do honest, reliable service on your car, you need someone you can trust to support and encourage you as you travel through life's traffic. A friend with whom you exercise can help you see your own progress when discouragement blindsides you. That same partner can motivate you to keep going that last 10 minutes to meet your goal! And, honestly, an exercise partner simply makes fitness more fun!

Maybe you have an exercise partner already, and you try to encourage yourself with affirmations. Things are going smoothly….until an illness or injury hits you! This is a negative that is out of your direct control, and it happens to everyone, elite athlete or recreational exerciser. Do not let it defeat your program. If you are sick, stop exercise until you are 24 hours past the last sign of your sickness, then start back cautiously until your strength has built back up. If you are injured, stop exercise with that body part until the pain goes away. Remember, an injury is not the same as a little muscle soreness from having a great workout. If you are a little sore the next day or two, but are able to carry out all of your daily activities without any problems, know that you are working hard and progress is happening. If the pain has not gone within 2 to 3 days, see a physician.

Both situations present a good time to schedule "NO exercise" in your appointment book, to help release the guilt and remind yourself that rest is important for your injury to heal. Your body will not begin losing significant fitness benefits from lack of activity until about two weeks have passed, and most illnesses and injuries do not exceed that length of time, right? You will need to return to your exercise program cautiously and conservatively, but your body will be right back where you left it within a week or so!

Your **FITNESS CHALLENGE** for Week 4: Perform a safety check by following the form and function guidelines during your next exercise session, noting any areas that need improvement. Secondly, look at the F.U.N. in your current exercise routine, and choose one strategy to put more flexibility, understanding, or positive reinforcement into your weekly exercise routine. **Record any safety changes and F.U.N. strategies in your Maintenance Log.**

A Look in the Rearview Mirror

Week 4: Tune Up

Foundation: Record at least three changes you have made on the Victory Lap chart (page 249) since Week 1, and reward yourself!

Food (Part 1): Choose at least three different snacks that will improve the quality of your carbohydrate fuel at your afternoon snack break.

Food (Part 2): Identify one of the "check the oil" challenges that you face and choose one step to improve the quality of your fat fuel.

Fitness: Improve one specific area under safety check and one under the F.U.N. strategies this week.

Now, record any changes you notice this week:

Date	Thoughts, Feelings, Body Changes?

PHASE TWO:
Let's Accelerate!

Week 5: Plan Your Pit Stops

Week 6: Charge Your Battery

Week 7: Clean the Rearview Mirror

Week 8: Deal with Detours

Week 5:

Plan Your Pit Stops

"People don't believe the weight battle I've had in the past (my whole life!) People always ask me how I remain thin in the restaurant business (I now own 2 Cheeburger Cheeburger restaurants in Louisiana and it is CRAZY!), and I tell them about Rev It Up!. Although my weight has fluctuated a little, I remain very close to the weight I was when I finished the program (over 2 years ago). I'm actually there now! I also wander off of the program occasionally (tired, stressed, eating at the restaurant every day, etc.) but ALWAYS come back to Rev It Up! and jump back in!"   Rebecca

Chapter 17

Plan Your Pit Stops:
Follow the Traffic Lights

You have spent a lot of time putting down a new foundation and meeting the challenges for all four "F's", including food, fluid, and fitness. You have taken the driver's seat and are revving up your metabolism-taking control-and noticing the difference. Now, the time has come to accelerate your focus-and begin fine-tuning your engine. Let's start Week 5 by turning our headlights on Food for an accelerated look at eating out-or, in Rev It Up! terms, PIT STOPS!

A *pit stop* for routine service or to refuel the engine is a common part of maintenance for any vehicle. Sometimes a pit stop may be required more frequently depending on the amount of driving or wear and tear on the vehicle. How does this translate to you and your metabolism? For Rev It Up! purposes, a *"Pit Stop" includes food you pick up, take out, eat out or that you purchase prepackaged.* Pit stops take you out of the controlled atmosphere of your home and put you at the mercy of someone else's menu or preparation. These stops may be even more frequent if you have a fast-paced schedule or are often on the road.

Did you know that the average person eats out at least one out of every three meals? Fast food restaurants with quick drive through windows make a pit stop easy. With "quick stop" food marts available on almost every corner, even a snack can be purchased in a matter of minutes. But choosing smart fuel or getting a quick paint job (fruits or vegetables!) can be very hard to do when your choices are high-fat foods that typically do not include color or whole grains.

What are some key strategies to take with you at any pit stop - fast food, quick stops or a sit-down restaurant? Learn the Traffic Lights to follow for your Pit Stops.

RED LIGHTS FOR PIT STOPS

1.   Don't go hungry! Watch your body's fuel gauge, and keep an eye on that clock. If you know you will be eating out for the next meal, make sure you plan for a snack in between meals if your body's fuel tank will have to wait longer than 4 hours. Making a pit stop BEFORE you reach a hunger level of 1 or 2 (you know, the "give me anything I can get my hands on...and quick!" levels!) will help control your cravings for fats or sugars. When you are able to think clearly and check the menu, you are more likely to select healthier food.

2.   Don't skip meals or neglect snacks! What's the problem with skipping a meal or snack, or two, to save up your calories to go splurge at one of your favorite restaurants? What may seem to make sense to you will not make sense to your body and its hunger and fullness cycle. Remember that your fuel tank holds about 4 hours of fuel at any given time, and if the tank is way beyond empty, you will most likely overeat. And when you overeat, any extra fuel that your body cannot use will need to be stored. Your body will be primed, ready and waiting to store the extra fuel as fat to prepare itself for the next time the pit stop is long overdue! So please, don't save up calories by skipping meals or snacks.

3.   Don't fill up on fast "fillers"! What sits on your table, tempting you to fill up before your meal even arrives? The bread or chip basket! It's hard to resist the warm smell of fresh baked bread or crispy chips. And a roll or a handful of chips can certainly be included as part of your grain portion. But too often, one baseball becomes 2 baseballs, maybe 3...even 4! And when the meal arrives, you are not physically hungry anymore but often eat most or all of your meal anyway because you are paying for it, or feel guilty and defeated and therefore assume "why not?" To stop filling up before the meal, choose one of the following strategies:

a.   Ask the wait staff to skip the bread or chip basket.
b.   Ask the wait staff to remove the bread or chip basket after you have selected a small amount.
c.   Ask the wait staff to bring the bread or chip basket to the table with your entrée to prevent filling up too early.

Okay, you are probably seeing enough "red" right now. Time to check out the green lights!

GREEN LIGHTS FOR PIT STOPS

1. Do save your ping pong balls! Don't save calories by skipping meals through the day, but you CAN save your fat servings (remember those three ping pong ball size portions?) for a meal at your favorite restaurant. Go ahead and eat balanced, but low- to no-fat, meals and snack on your regular schedule throughout the day. Save up most or all your ping pong ball amount of added fats for the restaurant meal. Your fat servings may all come at once, but your metabolism will not be slower and your cravings will be more controlled because you have eaten regularly throughout the day.

2. Do plan your splurges! When you arrive at a restaurant, decide on a "splurge" item and include it in your meal. Maybe your splurge is a dessert that you can share with the entire table. Or maybe you decide to share an extravagant entrée with a friend, and balance it by ordering a salad and a side order of vegetables. Assume that these special items will be cooked with fat for extra flavor; therefore, compromise in other areas that you can control. Ask for condiments like salad dressings "on the side" and skip the added butter on the bread. Limiting the added fats that you can control helps balance the special items that already have fat as part of the preparation. And if you continue to use the baseball guidelines to control your grain choices, the palm of your hand to control your protein, and look for ways to eat as much color as possible, you can still come out ahead AND enjoy yourself, too!

3. Do expand your expectations! You probably enjoy eating out for not only the food but also the atmosphere, the company with whom you are dining, and the night off from having to prepare a meal yourself. Expand your expectations of eating out to include the whole experience, and maybe the meal itself will take on a smaller role. This in turn can result in more attention to the event itself and less attention to finishing your plate.

4. Do drink your water! Restaurant or fast food meals typically contain more sodium (salt), used in the preparation, so drinking your water is an important strategy to help balance the higher sodium content. In addition, water is especially important if you consume alcohol at your meal. Alcohol will not only dehydrate you but also lower your resistance to food temptations and possibly increase your appetite at the same time. Remember to match up any alcohol you drink with an equal amount of additional water. This helps dilute the effect of the alcohol and ensures your body stays hydrated.

5.   Do remember "I can EAT AGAIN!" Once you eat your baseball amounts of grain, lots of color, and your palm sized portion of protein, ask the restaurant staff to bring a take-home box. Remember, you *can* eat it all, but listen to your fuel gauge when it tells you it's full, and eat the rest *later*!

Notice more green lights than red lights? Good! Eating out will remain a big part of our culture and can be incorporated into a healthy, well lifestyle with just a little more effort and planning. *Concentrate on the positive strategies and remember to take your Rev It Up! principles with you whenever you order a meal outside your home.* Don't leave home without them!

To help you make decisions about what fuel to order, take a look at the following list. It provides a guide to help you choose healthy options at a sit-down restaurant. The list is not comprehensive, but highlights common lower-fat options found in most restaurants.

Healthy Restaurant Fuel Choices

Appetizers:
Select items like tomato juice, broth-based hot or cold soups, or fresh fruit for a colorful start. Or choose shrimp cocktail, steamed mussels or an appetizer like pot stickers for more protein. Many restaurants will serve an appetizer portion of most entrées, which, along with a salad, can serve as your entire meal.

Salads:
Any mixed green salad is a great addition, and the deeper the green of the lettuces used, the better! Watch out for high-fat additions like

bacon, grated cheese, and croutons. And always request salad dressings on the side, so that you can control the amount used.

Entrées:

Lean cuts of beef or pork, roasted or grilled are great options. Also, roasted or grilled chicken, turkey or Cornish hen, with the skin removed, are excellent protein choices. And remember that broiled or grilled fish can help you meet your "check the oil" challenge to eat more omega 3 fatty acids. (NOTE: Many restaurants, particularly steakhouses, baste their beef, pork, poultry, and fish entrées with butter or oil. Ask if this is done, and if so, request that the chef eliminate this step.)   Other options include pasta entrées with tomato-based sauces or even vegetable pizza, with a thin or traditional style (not thick) crust.

Sides:

Any grilled, roasted, baked, boiled or steamed vegetable side dish helps add color to your meal. But avoid vegetables that are in a cream sauce (like creamed spinach or spinach dip), fried (like fried okra or potatoes) or in a casserole (like broccoli casserole). Grain type side dishes are always available, but note how they are prepared. A grain, like rice or risotto, is most often cooked in a cream or butter base. And many restaurants pour melted butter over their plain steamed vegetables, as well. So always ask how it is prepared if you do not know already, and keep an eye on portion control if the dish is made with added fats.

Desserts:

The lower-fat desserts are sorbet, sherbets and fruit-based choices. However, dessert is often a splurge, so you may opt to order a full-fat version but split it with several friends and/or take home the rest to share later.

Now you have a road map for sit-down restaurants. What about fast food options? Lately most if not all fast food restaurants have worked to bring at least a few healthy options for entrées and side items. The menu items can change, and some are regionally selective, but the following table will give you a head start on making healthy Rev It Up! choices for fast food pit stops:

Healthy Fast Food Fuel Choices

FAST FOOD	HEALTHY CHOICES	PORTION GUIDE 1 ppb = 1 ping pong ball (for fat serving)
Arby's	Roasted chicken sandwich, w/o mayo, side salad, *low-fat dressing	1 baseball of grain, palm size animal protein, 1 vegetable, 1 dairy protein (if cheese), 1 ppb fat*
	Regular roast beef sandwich w/ side salad, low-fat dressing (***use 1 ppb amount for all dressings**)	1 baseball of grain, palm size animal protein, 1 vegetable, 1 ppb fat*
	Grilled chicken salad, low-fat dressing*	palm size animal protein, 1 vegetable, 1 fruit, 1 ppb fat*
Burger King	Grilled chicken Whopper, w/ all the trimmings EXCEPT mayo, side salad w/ low-fat dressing*	1 ½ baseballs of grain, palm size animal protein, 1 vegetable, 1 ppb fat*
	Grilled chicken salad, w/ low-fat dressing*, and fruit side (if available)	palm size animal protein, 2 vegetables, (1 fruit), 1 ppb fat*
Chick-Fil-A	Grilled chicken deluxe sandwich, w/ small carrot raisin salad or fresh fruit	1 baseball of grain, palm size animal protein, vegetable and fruit combo
	Grilled or spicy chicken wrap, with low-fat dressing*	1 ½ baseball of grain, palm size animal protein, 1 vegetable, 1 ppb fat*

Chick-Fil-A (continued)	Grilled chicken salad w/ low-fat dressing*, carrot raisin or fruit salad	Palm size animal protein, 2 vegetables, 1 fruit, 1 ppb fat*

KFC	BBQ chicken sandwich, side of green beans* (fat added in cooking)	1 baseball of grain, palm size animal protein, 1 vegetable, 1 ppb fat
	Grilled chicken breast (no skin) w/ mashed potatoes (no gravy), green beans*	1 baseball of grain, palm size animal protein, 1 vegetable, 1 ppb fat*
McDonald's	Grilled chicken sandwich, w/o mayo (ask for extra lettuce & tomato), apples	1 baseball of grain, palm size animal protein,1 vegetable, 1 fruit
	Grilled chicken salad, without bacon, w/ low-fat dressing*, apple slices	palm size animal protein, 1 dairy protein, 2 vegetables, 1 ppb fat*
	Grilled chicken snack wrap, no sauce, apple slices	1 baseball of grain, ½ palm size animal and dairy protein (combo), 1 fruit
Subway	Any of the "6 grams of fat or less" sandwich options, loaded with fresh veggies (6" size); vinegar optional, apple slices or raisins	2 baseballs of grain, palm size animal protein, 2 vegetable, (1 dairy protein if cheese included), fruit

Taco Bell	Two soft chicken tacos	1 ½ baseballs of grain, palm size animal protein, 1 vegetable, 1 dairy protein
	Taco salad without the hard shell, with salsa as dressing	1 baseball grain (beans), palm size animal protein, 2 vegetables, 1 dairy protein
Wendy's	Baked potato (no butter / sour cream), stuffed with chili, and garden salad w/ low-fat dressing*	2 baseballs of grain, palm size animal/ plant protein (chili), 2 vegetables, 1 ppb fat*
	Bowl of chili, garden salad, w/ low-fat dressing*	1 baseball of grain, palm size animal/ plant protein (in chili), 2 vegetables, 1 ppb fat*
	Grilled chicken sandwich (no sauce), garden salad w/ low-fat dressing*	1 baseball of grain, palm size animal protein, 2 vegetable, 1 ppb fat*
	Mandarin chicken salad (w/ almonds, noodles*, oranges), w/ ½ pack oriental sesame dressing*	1 baseball grain, palm size animal/ plant protein, 2 vegetables, 1/2 fruit, 1 ½ ppb fat*

Although this list is not comprehensive, hopefully it will help you make a more informed decision about where and what to eat. The portion guidelines are specifically based on the food items listed in the middle column compared to the calorie calculations provided by each restaurant; therefore, the portions listed may or may not meet your individual goal so adjust accordingly. If you do choose to have the traditional fast food meal of a hamburger and French fries, just try not to "super size" and listen to your body's fuel gauge for fullness. Remember that *balance is the key* and one high-fat meal will not slow down your progress. It is what you do *more often than not* that will make the long term difference and promote a revved up metabolism.

Healthy pit stops can help you stay on track. But what about those times when you are hungry but unable to stop at a restaurant or even drive through for fast food? Two of the most common situations are when you are <u>driving</u> or when you are <u>flying</u>.

The strategies that follow will help you prepare for the next time you might be on a long trip in the car or an airplane, heading towards an empty fuel gauge but unable to stop to refuel.

REV IT UP WHEN YOU ARE DRIVING:

1.   Carry a small cooler with an ice pack inside and include foods such as fresh fruit, baby carrots, drinkable low-fat yogurt, and string cheese.

2.   Stash some high-energy treats in the glove compartment, such as energy bars (Choose the flavors that will not melt! See Question #13 in "Most Frequently Asked Questions" in the Appendix for more information on energy bars). Other options include dried fruits like raisins, single serving whole grain cereal boxes, small snack bags of nuts and pretzels, or nuts and cereal mix (home made is preferable).

3.   Take the smart approach at a gas station pit stop-purchase a water bottle and a healthier snack option like raisins, pretzels, or a cereal bar. Having a hard time resisting a candy bar? Choose a miniature "feel good" treat like a peppermint patty or several chocolate kisses instead. Savor the treat on the road by seeing how long you can make the chocolate last. You may find that a little bit can go a long way in satisfaction if you slow down enough to really enjoy it.

Staying on track with your fuel stops while driving is easier than when flying, but you can use the following guidelines to help you:

REV IT UP WHEN YOU ARE FLYING:

1.   Carry snacks with you in your briefcase or purse, such as dried fruit, home made trail mix in a throwaway container (try oat cereal with raisins and almond slices), or natural peanut butter crackers. And don't forget to purchase a water bottle right before stepping on the plane.

2.   Drink extra water at every opportunity. This is the perfect time to match up those fluids, since airplane travel automatically limits the availability of water and takes more water out of your body naturally.

3.   Check to see if your flight provides meals or snacks. Don't get caught in a time change and miss the opportunity to purchase a meal to carry with you if the flight does not provide it. Healthy options are available now in most terminal restaurants, and if all else fails, simply get a slice of cheese pizza to take on the plane (a bit messier, but it works in a pinch). Since color options are few and far between, try to plan and pack individual snack size bags of raw carrots, or individual boxes of dried fruit.

4.   Do the best you can! Don't worry if you get caught in the rush of traveling and forget to pack snacks or somehow miss a meal. Simply do what you can with what you have…and get right back on track when you arrive. Start by purchasing a water bottle and small bag of nuts once your plane lands, and enjoy these while waiting for your luggage. If your fuel gauge is running on empty, this snack will carry you through the taxi or bus ride to your next stop.

NOTE: *Now that you are in the Acceleration phase of Rev It Up!, you no longer have four separate challenges for Foundation, Food, Fluid, and Fitness. Your weekly challenge will concentrate on only ONE of the Four "F's", and will be found on the "Look in the Rearview Mirror" page after each chapter.*

A Look in the Rearview Mirror

Week 5: Plan Your Pit Stops

Your **ACCELERATION Challenge** for Week 5: Choose healthy options when you make a pit stop this week. Remember, pit stops include restaurant meals, fast food, and take-out foods.

Now, record any changes you notice this week:

Date	Thoughts, Feelings, Body Changes?

Week 6:

Charge Your Battery

"I have found two benefits from the exercise part of the program: 1) You lose inches, and 2) You get more compliments! I have a dress that I wore to my nephew's wedding. I haven't really lost any weight since I wore it last August, but it was pretty form fitting. I wore it yesterday to Easter services and it is now loose-so I guess that as much as I do not like the gym work, it's good for me!

Today I also saw an eye doctor that I had not seen before, so he doesn't know what I used to look like, and he asked me if I played tennis, because I looked really fit! The other cool part was that I had decided to get new frame- the ones I had are outdated and are bigger than the current style-but in addition to that they are now much too big looking for my much thinner face!"   Beth

Chapter 18

Battery Charge
Using Aerobic Exercise

Whether a fitness plan was something new to you or you were already working out when you started Rev It Up!, over the past weeks you have started taking your body to the next level. Hopefully you are seeing the benefits of a stronger heart and stronger muscles in everyday life.

When you first started your exercise plan, or as you increased the amount and type of exercise you were already doing, this new level produced initial results that you could see and feel. You may still be seeing steady benefits, and your body does not need a battery charge just yet. But, you will inevitably hit a fitness plateau sometime in the future as your body adjusts to its new routine. In fact, you may already have noticed that the benefits you first obtained seem to have lessened over time. And you are getting discouraged. If you are, what can you do to stop this plateau from happening? Learn how to *charge your battery* using both types of fitness to make the most of your efforts over the long haul.

Have you ever experienced the frustration of trying to start your car, but discover no response? Your battery is dead! The only way to correct the problem is to charge it up again. Likewise, if you feel your exercise is lacking energy or not getting the results now that you noticed when you first started, charge your battery!

BATTERY CHARGE USING AEROBIC EXERCISE

A battery charge, using aerobic exercise, requires changing the intensity of your aerobic workout. At what level of intensity will you receive the most benefit from your exercise? In other words, how do you keep your battery charged for the most efficient performance? Three strategies to try are as follows:

Strategy #1: Exercise at a steady rate but a HIGHER intensity level during the entire workout.

Strategy #2: Alternate higher bursts of intense activity with periods of recovery during the same workout.

Strategy #3: Use correct form while you exercise on equipment like a treadmill, stair climber or an elliptical trainer.

STRATEGY #1:

Exercise at a STEADY rate but HIGHER INTENSITY level

During any type of physical activity, your body gets its fuel from both fat and stored carbohydrate, called glycogen, found in your muscles and your liver. If you exercise at a lower intensity, say, 65% of your target heart rate, your body prefers to use more of its fat stores and less of its glycogen stores. If you exercise at a higher intensity, say 80 to 85% of your target heart rate, your body draws more energy from your glycogen, or carbohydrate, stores instead of your fat stores. Does this mean that lower-intensity exercise is better? Not necessarily! The key is not the type of fuel you burn but the amount that you burn that charges your battery most efficiently. Let's look at an example:

Scenario A: *45 minutes* of exercise time, *lower* intensity

Joe works out for 45 minutes at 65% of his target heart rate and burns a total of 350 calories. About 50% of the total calories burned are fat, so Joe burned about 175 calories from his fat stores in 45 minutes.

Scenario B: *Same amount* of exercise time, but *moderate* intensity

Joe works out for 45 minutes at about 75% of his target heart rate and burns a total of 500 calories. About 40% of his total calories burned are fat, so Joe burned about 200 calories from his fat stores. Increasing the intensity resulted in more calories burned from his fat stores than working out at a lower intensity, even in the same amount of time.

Scenario C: *Less* exercise time, but *highest* intensity

Joe works out for 30 minutes only, but at about 80 to 85% of his target heart rate and burns a total of 500 calories. About 35% of his total calories burned are fat, so Joe burned about 175 calories from his fat stores. Increasing the intensity even more resulted in the same number of calories burned from his fat stores as did the lowest intensity workout but in *less* time!

Did you notice what happened? Compare the first and second scenarios. When Joe worked out for the *same* amount of time, but at different intensity levels (harder), he not only burned *more* calories but also a little more body *fat*, even though the total % of calories burned from fat was less. Compare this to the third scenario, when Joe actually worked out *less* time but at the highest intensity level. He burned more calories and the same amount of fat as in the first scenario but in only 30 minutes, saving 15 minutes. This can come in handy when your own exercise time is limited. So learn from Joe and take advantage of a battery charge by increasing the intensity of your workout within your target heart rate range.

Just in case you do not remember your target heart rate (THR) range, look back in Chapter 8 on page 89. You can continue to use that formula, or you can incorporate your resting heart rate (RHR) into the formula that follows. This formula, called the Karvonen Method, is more individualized and accurate, especially for someone who has been exercising regularly for awhile. But the key is to know your resting heart rate. Once you have your RHR, you subtract that number from a standard maximum heart rate for males or females, then you add the RHR number back into the equation after multiplying by the intensity level. Work this out step by step:

KARVONEN TARGET HEART RATE FORMULA:

Determine your average resting heart rate (RHR) by taking your pulse rate (hold the count for 60 seconds) immediately upon waking, before rising from bed. Record, and repeat this for three days. Determine your average RHR by multiplying the three days' numbers together and dividing by three; RHR = _____

For males:

(220 – RHR_____)x 65% + RHR = _____ (Lowest THR)

(220 – RHR_____)x 85% + RHR = _____ (Highest THR)

For females:

(226 – RHR_____)x 65% + RHR = _____ (Lowest THR)

(226 – RHR_____)x 85% + RHR = _____ (Highest THR)

You can now divide these two final numbers by 6 to determine what a 10 second heart rate count is for you:

Lowest THR _____) ÷ 6 = _____ (lowest 10 sec count)
Highest THR_____) ÷ 6 = _____ (highest 10 sec count)

STRATEGY #2:
ALTERNATE higher bursts of activity
with periods of recovery

Do you want to try another approach to increase intensity? Alternate bursts of intense activity *several times* during the same workout instead of just staying at the same intensity level, albeit higher, during the entire workout. This concept is known as **interval training**.

For example, increase your intensity on the treadmill to the upper limit of your target heart rate zone (80 to 85%, or the "I can't talk now!" zone) after about 5 to 10 minutes of warming up your muscles and hold this highest intensity for 1 to 2 minutes. Then reduce the intensity back to 65% of your target heart rate and recover 2 to 4 minutes. Repeat this *burst and recovery* pattern (in which you have a 1:2 ratio for the amount of time at the intense level and the amount of recovery time, respectively) during the entire exercise time, allowing for about a 10-minute cool-down before stopping exercise. If your health history allows, you can take this concept one step further and increase your intensity above your target heart rate zone (85% to 90%). Hold this level for 15 to 30 seconds, followed by about 2 minutes of recovery, allowing your heart rate to return to 65%, the lower intensity target heart rate zone.

Another way to incorporate interval training is varying the aerobic machines during the same workout period. For example, after warming up, work 10 minutes on the treadmill, then immediately switch to the elliptical trainer for the next 15 minutes, followed by a final 10 minutes on a stationary cycle. Return to the treadmill for your 5-minute cool-down. Changing machines changes the muscles worked, and your body stays more "alert" in the process.

Is there a beneficial difference between interval training or simply increasing intensity at a steady rate? Both certainly rev up your metabolism, and both will encourage your body to continue to burn calories at a higher rate for a period of time after the exercise is over. But the interval training gives you the longest after-burn effect and trains your body to recover more quickly. Even if your burst and recovery pattern is irregular or at different durations of time, you will see your body benefit. For example, you may choose to maintain high intensity for 3 or 4 minutes and recover for the same amount of time, or your bursts may be as short as 60 seconds. Get creative. Burst when you feel like it and slow down when your body tells you, even if the time periods don't fit a pattern. You WILL see a difference!

STRATEGY #3:
Use CORRECT FORM while exercising

If you enjoy exercising on the treadmill, stair climber or elliptical machine, here is a hint that will help you get the most out of your workout time...*let go of the handles!* Research has proven that holding the handrails of an exercise machine while you work out reduces your heart rate and the amount of oxygen consumed. Your body will not burn the amount of calories that it should burn if you hold on, unless the equipment itself is designed to include movable arm handles for an upper *and* lower body workout.

You may not feel secure increasing the speed or the elevation without holding onto the handrails at the same time. But part of the challenge itself is the balance required to do the activity. You may need to decrease the speed at which you normally work when you first let go. And make sure you do not increase the speed or elevation too quickly-only small increments at a time. Too high a speed or pace will probably force you to hold on, and holding on at high speeds can lead to serious back or knee injuries because it requires you to rotate your hips to an incorrect angle. *Just make sure that you do not increase the speed or elevation too quickly-only small increments at a time.*

On that same thought, keep your head aligned with your spine, keep your shoulders relaxed and hold in your stomach muscles to maintain correct form. Once you have adjusted to letting go, readjusted your speed and feel comfortable again, challenge your body by maintaining that speed but gradually adding elevation or resistance in small increments. The next week, maintain your speed and elevation and add a little more time or distance, like an extra ¼ mile. Regardless of what change you make, you are charging your body's battery and improving your balance at the same time.

Chapter 19

Battery Charge
Using Strength Training

Charging your battery by aerobic exercise depends on the level of intensity of your workout. What about charging your battery using strength training? The key is to develop both muscle strength and muscle endurance. You can develop both of these, strength and endurance, by using the following principles to charge your battery for strength training:

Strategy #1: Overload your muscles using resistance, frequency and duration for each movement.

Strategy #2: Change the amount of rest between exercise.

Strategy #3: Switch movements for the same muscle group.

STRATEGY #1:

OVERLOAD your muscles

Overload in strength training is a good thing. It happens when the resistance (amount of weight), the frequency (how many times it happens) or the duration (how long it continues) increases. You can do this by changing the amount of weight (resistance), changing the number of sets of each exercise (frequency) or changing the amount of time it takes to do the exercise (duration). Using bicep curls as an example, let's look at ways that you can put this principle to work for you:

RESISTANCE: Let's say that you can comfortably lift a 5 pound dumbbell for 3 sets of 12 repetitions each (that's 36 times!). It is now time to charge your battery and one way to do this is to add resistance. Increase the amount of weight to an 8 pound dumbbell. However, when you increase the weight load, you need to automatically decrease the number of times you lift it at first. Work your way back up as you gain strength.

FREQUENCY: As you progress, you can add one or two repetitions for each set over a period of weeks until you can comfortably lift 3 sets of 12 repetitions.

DURATION: Adding repetitions naturally adds to the time each set will take, increasing the duration of the exercise. Another way to extend the duration is do the repetition even slower-try four counts up and four counts down. Once you can complete 3 sets of 12 repetitions, for a longer duration, it is time to overload again.

STRATEGY #2:

CHANGE the amount of REST between exercises

In your current routine, you may complete your 3 sets of bicep exercises, rest between each set, and start your triceps exercises. Instead, why don't you perform 1 set of bicep curls, follow this with 1 set of tricep kick-backs, follow by repeating the bicep curls, then complete another set of tricep kick-backs? Continue until you have completed three sets of each, and then rest. You can alternate an exercise for the bicep with a movement for the tricep because you are working complementary or opposite muscle groups. This routine takes the greatest advantage of your time and challenges your muscles to be stronger and endure longer.

STRATEGY #3:

SWITCH MOVEMENTS for the same muscle group

Pump up the intensity of your workout by doing the same exercise, but in a more challenging way. For example, if you have been doing sit-ups or abdominal curls with your hands resting behind your head, try to rev it up by extending your arms further behind your head when you do this exercise. Be careful to keep your shoulders as relaxed as possible, and keep the lower back pressed to the floor. You will probably need to decrease the number of repetitions in the beginning and work your way back up.

Another example uses push ups. If you have been doing this exercise with your knees and lower legs on the floor, try a more challenging position. Do them with only your knees on the floor and your lower legs lifted. Or extend your legs with only your feet and hands supporting your body. Keep your back straight and lift your body using only your chest and arm strength. This is the hardest way, but you can build your strength by reducing the number of sets and repetitions in the beginning, and work up to the full count again.

Or try doing your bicep curls and tricep kick-backs while sitting on a flex ball. The motions are the same, but your body has to ask your abdominal muscles to help balance you on the flex ball. The more muscles you are working at any given moment, the more benefit you receive. You are strengthening your core at the same time you are building upper body strength. It's a win-win situation!

Time to *take some action*! With any change in exercise, a record of your progress can be very encouraging and reminds you how you are improving your fitness week by week. Take a minute and complete the following:

Record any current exercises that are easy for you:

Aerobic exercise: _____   _____

_____

Strength training exercise: _____

_____

Next, choose one of the strategies below to charge your fitness battery for each type of exercise:

Increase the intensity of your aerobic workout by:

1.   Increasing your heart rate within your target range and holding this new level for the duration of the activity.

2.   Alternating bursts of intensity with periods of recovery by repeatedly increasing your heart rate to 85% of your target range for 1 to 2 minutes followed by recovering your heart rate back to 65% for 2 to 4 minutes.

3.   Letting go of the handrails (probably will need to reduce the intensity at first!) to challenge not only your heart but also your balance.

Increase the intensity of your strength training by:

1.   Overloading your muscles during your workout.

2.   Changing the amount of rest between your exercises

3.   Switching movements for the same muscle group.

Now, finish the following sentence, filling in one or more of these strategies: *I will charge my fitness battery using each type of exercise in the following new way*:

Aerobic exercise: _____

_____

Strength training: _____

_____

Finally, do it THIS WEEK!

A Look in the Rearview Mirror

Week 6: Charge Your Battery

Your **ACCELERATION Challenge** for Week 6:   Charge your battery by choosing one strategy to increase the intensity of your aerobic activity on 2 of the 4 days and/or one strategy to increase the intensity of your strength training on 1 of the 2 days. Highlight the days that you use these strategies in your Maintenance Log.

Now, record any changes you notice this week:

Date	Thoughts, Feelings, Body Changes?

Week 7:

Clean the Rearview Mirror

"The most beneficial part of Rev It Up! has been feeling good about myself and healthy in my own body. Knowing that being healthy at this point in my life is more important than being skinny."   Sandy

"It has been one year since I started Rev It Up!. To date I have lost around 35 pounds and 30 inches. Can't really do the size thing, because I have changed size ranges-no more "W's" at the end of the size I wear! I was on the beach last week in a bathing suit and just a cover-up and was not self-conscious about the way I looked. Thanks again for teaching me how to do this!"   Elizabeth

Chapter 20

Clean Your Mirror
to Improve Your View

Pit stops, battery charges....can you hear your engine accelerating as a result of your new choices? The changes you have focused on these last two weeks have been external choices-what you actually order from a restaurant menu, or what combination of aerobic machines you choose at the gym. You've been looking on the outside-it's time to stop and turn your headlights inward. Are your thoughts about yourself matching up with the changes you are making on the outside?

Picture this: You enter the doors of your gym for a workout, feeling proud of yourself that you have made time to exercise. As you walk towards a treadmill, you begin noticing the gentleman lifting heavy weights, the lady running on another treadmill nearby, and the aerobic instructor heading to class. Your biceps do not look like that guy, your pace cannot even keep up with your neighbor's, and the aerobics instructor must not have an ounce of fat on her legs! All of a sudden, you do not feel so proud of yourself, decide to shorten your workout time and head home.

What happened? Your body image has entered the picture, and it's not a reflection you like. How you see your body and how you think others see your body greatly affects how you feel about yourself. And how you feel about your body cannot be separated from how you treat that very same body...the fuel you give it and the activity you ask it to do.

A positive body image does not necessarily mean that you love everything about your body and have no need or desire to make any changes. It *does* mean that you have a healthy self identity, can appreciate the positive things that your body can do, and can enjoy life for the moment instead of waiting until you reach a certain weight.

Do you struggle with a negative body image? "Look in the mirror" and see how you answer the following:

Yes No   Body Image Test

___ ___ • Your mood can change immediately if someone comments on your clothes, your looks, or your body.

___ ___ • You catch a glimpse of yourself in the mirror and only notice what you do not like about your body.

___ ___ • You refuse to accept a compliment from someone, and often negate the remark or criticize yourself in some way.

___ ___ • You frequently ask your family or friends if you look okay.

___ ___ • You believe that if you can just lose a certain number of pounds or wear a certain size that you will feel better about yourself.

___ ___ • You frequently criticize other people's bodies or clothing, or looks.

___ ___ • You frequently make excuses to avoid a social event because you feel fat or do not like your appearance.

___ ___ • You punish yourself by not allowing yourself to eat certain foods because they are "bad."

___ ___ • You exercise only to burn calories in an effort to try to lose weight or burn off excess calories you consumed in a previous meal.

___ ___ • You fixate on a certain body part you do not like rather than concentrate on your body or appearance as a whole.

Enter the total of your 'Yes' and 'No' answers:
Yes _____   **No** _____
If you answered yes to five or more, your negative body image has strong influences over your level of health and wellness.

So what can you do? Where do you start to make a change from a negative to a positive body image? Check the mirror and notice what you see. Does it reflect the *real you* or is the image distorted? It's time to *clean your mirror* to improve your reflection.

When you drive your car, you depend on your mirror to see behind you, in order to drive safely and with purpose. You also need your mirror to be clean, not cloudy or broken. Only a mirror free of dirt or broken glass can give the driver a true reflection of the situation. And regardless of the condition of the mirror, you cannot look in your mirror constantly and continue to move forward. You must look away from the mirror to concentrate on the road ahead. In fact, most of your driving requires a steady look ahead with just an occasional glimpse in the mirror's reflection.

Likewise, your body's image is the reflection you see in your mirror. The mirror often reflects what is in your past, behind you, and includes images that have been developed throughout your life. These images are influenced by things you have heard, read, and seen. Over time, dirt may have accumulated and it affects how clearly you can see what is really happening. Or your body image might even be broken from years of abuse or neglect. Do you spend more time looking back in the mirror's reflection, unaware that it's broken or dirty and distorts the picture you see?

To move forward, you need to clean and repair your mirror, or body image, *and stay focused on the road before you instead of the path behind you.* This can take a lot of time and patience, but the rewards of a clear reflection help guarantee more security and confidence as you keep your eyes on the road ahead. So let's see what it takes to clean your mirror. In other words, change your body image.

First, believe that your body is capable of change. Remind yourself about all the things you have changed already like drinking more water, eating more colors, listening to your hunger cues, or eating every four hours. Next, believe that change happens one small step at a time. No need to feel that change must happen overnight to be successful. It's a process that takes time. Finally, believe that your body image does not have to be limited to body weight changes only. Body image changes include how we relate to other people, how much we allow our thoughts about our body to affect our moods, and how we interact socially.

True change cannot be rooted in external changes that work only as a temporary Band-aid to cover up the problem, but must be rooted from the inside out. To be successful in body image change, you need to *own* your own body and its ability to change. Begin implementing and maintaining these changes as an ongoing lifestyle, not without setbacks but always without judgment.

Are you ready to clean your mirror, and begin seeing a new reflection? Try one of the following strategies:

Clean Your Mirror for a New Reflection

1. *Think about someone you admire and respect.* Describe the characteristics of this person that you most admire:

    _____

    _____

    _____

    Don't be surprised if appearance is *not* one of the top priorities that you list when describing characteristics you respect!

2. *List 5 physical strengths about your body as a whole.* For example, "my legs are strong..." or "my smile is engaging..."

    _____

    _____

    _____

3. *Make a list of positive statements about your body that emphasize the way you want to think about yourself.* For example, "my body deserves to be nurtured by food"...or... "I can enjoy a day at the pool regardless of my swimsuit size."

_____

_____

_____

Repeat this list to yourself at least once in the morning and once in the evening. You do not have to feel or believe any of these positive statements as you say them, but you do need to repeat them. Just like hearing a song on the radio repetitively until you notice that one day you know every word without even trying-and that same song runs through your head all the time-new words, positive statements, that you repeat frequently can begin covering up the old reflections of your body and replacing it with a more nurturing one.

4. *Avoid magazines, television shows, or movies that make you feel bad about yourself* or only present the impossible as a role model.

5. Make an effort to *avoid criticizing other people* about their weight, clothes, or looks. If you comment on that person, limit it to positive comments about who they are or something they do, not how they look.

6. Look around when you are in a grocery store or in a department store and *notice that everyday people in your life come in ALL shapes and sizes.* Their bodies are more realistic than the models in the magazines.

7. Commit yourself to *view exercise as an opportunity to enjoy the movement of your body* and enjoy the experience itself. Notice how your body breathes, how your muscles work, and how your stress level decreases after you cool down.

8. *Begin eliminating your good/bad food list.* All foods have a place in your life, but become aware of how different foods affect your energy and your overall wellness. If you crave a gourmet chocolate chip cookie, you will not be satisfied by substituting a fat-free

alternative. But if that chocolate chip cookie is on your "bad" list, then you automatically become a "bad person" by eating it. Get rid of the moral judgments surrounding food! You are so much more than what you eat! To remove the craving, it may be best to simply indulge in one of those cookies, but eliminate other distractions, sit, and slowly enjoy every bite. And then just *move on*! Your craving will be satisfied without having to eat more calories from other alternatives that are not what you really wanted in the first place.

9. Notice what words you use to describe yourself and *do not allow yourself to select negative descriptions about your size or shape*. If you catch yourself criticizing your appearance, follow that with a positive comment about your body or looks or even your efforts to make a difference in how you view yourself.

10. Whenever you are tempted to concentrate on only one body part that you do not like, *remind yourself to look at the whole picture*. Remember that you do not compartmentalize other people that you respect and admire; so do yourself the same favor.

Hopefully this list of strategies for cleaning your mirror provides a starting place for a new body image. Regardless, realize that old dirt and cracks are hard to remove, so be patient and kind to yourself as you create a new reflection. You won't look in the mirror the same way again!

A Look in the Rearview Mirror

Week 7: Clean the Rearview Mirror

Your **ACCELERATION Challenge** for Week 7: Write down at least two positive statements and/or physical strengths about your own body, and display this list in a location that is privately accessible to you. Read this list at least twice a day, preferably in the morning after rising and in the evening before going to sleep.

Now, record any changes you notice this week:

Date	Thoughts, Feelings, Body Changes?

Week 8:

Deal With Detours

"Most definitely Rev It Up! has been a positive influence on my life. It taught me self-control and the means to achieve the body and health I wanted. Even when I 'mess up' with my eating, I know that it doesn't mean I've failed. I just get over it and begin again."   Becky

Chapter 21

Four Detours that Block Your Road

Last week was not easy. Cleaning those mirrors can be very exhausting, especially if they have years of dirt and grime. Your efforts will pay off-don't give up-because a clear view in your rearview mirror will guarantee less stress and more focus as you travel. In the meantime, since your headlights are already focused internally, let's take a good, hard look at the detours in your life.

Imagine this scenario: You are driving along, your tank has plenty of gas, and your car is running great. You have planned your time well, and traffic is minimal. You expect to reach your destination with a few minutes to spare. But what you *don't* expect is waiting for you right around the next corner...a DETOUR SIGN!

Often when you think things are running smoothly, you'll reach a fork in the road, pointing the way to a detour on an alternative road that may or may not be familiar to you. Detours can take you out of the way of your destination, but if you remain calm and patient, and stay alert, you will find your way back. You might lose some time, but *you do not have to lose your way*.

What detours do you run across most often on your road to a revved up metabolism? Is it the Detour of **SPECIAL EVENTS**, the Detour of **SIGHTS, SOUNDS, AND SMELLS**, the Detour of **PEOPLE PRESSURES**, or the Detour of **EMOTIONS**? Take a closer look at each one, and let's find new directions to follow to get us back on track.

The DETOUR of SPECIAL EVENTS

Are you able to follow your hunger and fullness cues, and choose smart fuel choices, UNLESS:

- You are on vacation?
- It's a holiday?

- You are at the movies?
- You are attending a sports event?
- It's your birthday party?
- It's your friend's birthday party?
- For that matter, it's the second cousin of your friend's former neighbor's birthday party?
- Basically, it's ANY PARTY?

Certainly special occasions like your birthday, Thanksgiving, or other holidays are times to celebrate, and a celebration usually includes an abundance of foods. Likewise, a vacation from work or routines can trigger a vacation from healthy food choices and exercise as well. In fact, a movie or a baseball game may even qualify for a "mini" special event or vacation. Do movie theaters trigger the need for a super-sized soda and large buttered popcorn, even if you have just eaten a meal? Does a sporting event, like a baseball game, trigger the desire for a foot-long hot dog and order of curly fries? Every time? Regardless of whether you are hungry or not? Does a vacation on the beach go hand in hand with several trips down that famous seafood buffet line-to try everything even if you feel more stuffed than the flounder entrée you just ate?

If you answered "yes" to two or more of these questions, a special event detour may force you to take an unexpected left or right turn more often than you realize.

The DETOUR of SIGHTS, SOUNDS, and SMELLS:

Ahhhh, the aroma of fresh baked cinnamon rolls…the crunch of potato chips resounding from your office's break room…the sight of brownie á la mode on a nearby restaurant table…the smell of barbecue on a hot summer day…even the sight of an advertisement in a magazine for Mrs. Field's chocolate chip cookies. Do these sights, sounds, and smells trigger an automatic "I must have these…now!" response, regardless of whether you are really hungry *or* whether it is time to refuel your tank or not?

It is not just coincidence that your local grocery store greets you with its bakery's smells and sights. And the big pictures of all the fast food combos at the drive-through window are not printed just to fill up space. These are designed to take advantage of your sight, sound and smell triggers…and hopefully trigger a bigger sale, and, therefore, a bigger profit!

Enjoying the sights, sounds, and smells of great food is part of the eating experience. However, if these things cause you to lose your direction often, and eat *just because*, you may want to look closer at this detour.

STRATEGIES for DETOURS 1 and 2

These first two detours, SPECIAL EVENTS and SIGHTS, SOUNDS AND SMELLS, often overlap each other; therefore, the strategies for dealing with these are similar. Stay alert, and you'll be more aware and on the lookout for the frequent warning signs of an upcoming detour. Then try the following strategies:

1.   First of all, know which trigger causes you the most difficulty.
2.   Be on the lookout for early warning signs.
3.   Don't arrive hungry-keep an eye on your body's fuel gauge to make sure you aren't in the middle of a detour when your gas tank is empty.
4.   Plan ahead and know your options.
5.   Have an escape plan.

Here are some "escape plans" to consider:

A)   **AT THE MOVIES:** If you must indulge in movie popcorn whenever you go to a movie theater, try the following:

- Send someone else to purchase the smallest size so that you are not tempted to order "super size, with extra butter please!"

- Plan to share your popcorn with a friend or family.

- Try to eat a few kernels at a time, instead of grabbing and eating a handful each time you reach into the bag. (This one sounds so simple but can be so hard! Make it a game to see how long you can make the kernels last-going for the length of the entire movie!)

B)   AT THANKSGIVING DINNER WITH GRANDMA: If you look forward to grandmother's famous sweet potato casserole at Thanksgiving, plan ahead. Don't miss the chance to have some, but stay in alignment with your meal and snack portions. Look at what is being offered to eat. Foods like hard rolls or buttered corn can be had at any time, but grandmother's casserole is a family holiday tradition. Choose it over the "nothing special" options, and savor each bite to maximize your enjoyment without over fueling your tank. You can skip the calories from the roll and the corn-grandmother's recipe is worth it!

C)   AT THE ANNUAL HOLIDAY PARTY: In this situation, your escape plan begins with a survey-*survey the buffet!* Look over all of the foods offered *before* putting the first bite in your mouth or on your plate. Have fried shrimp every year, but you've never tasted the stuffed crab? Eat brownies countless of times, but you rarely have an opportunity to enjoy your co-worker's famous chocolate candy? Choose two or three items that are "must have's", and fill up the rest of your plate with fresh fruit, crisp veggies, lots of color. Then move away from the buffet table, sit down, and savor every bite of those select items, nibbling on fruit and veggies to fill in the gap. You have made special choices, so you won't feel deprived, and you've survived a buffet without stuffing yourself! You made it through the detour's twists and turns and are on the road again.

D)   AT THE MALL: If you are in a situation where the sight of food is just too hard to ignore, consider purchasing it but plan to take it with you to enjoy later. For example, you are window-shopping in the local mall and smell fresh cinnamon rolls from the vendor nearby. You *must* have one!

- Purchase one, but ask to have it packaged to go and get away from the environment of the immediate sights and smells.
- Wait a few minutes, maybe by distracting yourself within another store. When you are not in the trigger's territory, you will have a chance to think more clearly. "Am I really hungry now? When did I last fuel my body?"

Be satisfied with the fact that you *own* that food item now. But make a decision based on your body's needs instead of your trigger's temptation. Don't forget the "I can eat again!" power. Save the treat for when you are really hungry and your fuel gauge is low. You might even find out that the cinnamon roll doesn't look or taste as appealing when it has been allowed to cool and harden. You don't know for sure, but it's worth a try. Now time to move on to another common problem...

The DETOUR of PEOPLE PRESSURES:

Do you have a friend or a family member who seems to always encourage you to eat "just another bite" or "try at least one?" What about the family member who trained you as a child to eat every last morsel of food on your plate because of the starving children in another country? Granted, children are starving all over the world, but eating everything on your plate probably did not help them in any way at that moment. But you still hear the voice of that relative each time you sit down to a meal.

What about someone who not only persuades you to eat even when you are not hungry but also acts hurt if you do not eat as much as they do? Or maybe your distant cousin, a great cook, claims that you must not like her food when you say no to the second helping at your annual family reunion. This detour is difficult, because your decision to eat or not to eat involves food AND relationships!

Your strategy is to identify the pressure. Once you have identified the people who create the pressure, you can better plan how to handle them. The following strategies are divided into a Relationship Option and a Reaction Option. Consider putting at least one of these into action:

STRATEGY for DETOUR 3

RELATIONSHIP OPTION:

Sometimes the situation will lead to the chance to talk to the people in your life who pressure you. Try to:

1.   Spend some time thinking about your friends and family, and distinguish who supports you and who pressures you.

2.   After you share your new understanding about your metabolism and your commitment to listen to your body with the person who pressures you, ask for his or her support of your new way of eating.

3.   Engage the person who pressures you as a Rev It Up! partner and challenge him or her to start listening to the body's own fuel gauge and see what happens!

REACTION OPTION:

Sometimes you are not able to discuss the situation with the people in your life due to the lack of opportunity or simply not feeling confident enough to do so. If this is the situation, concentrate on changing your reaction:

1.   Recommit yourself to listen to your body instead of listening to the person's pressure to eat when you are not hungry.

2.   Reconsider the results of your actions. Although you may feel subconscious pressure from the childhood memory of being told to "always clean your plate," doing so does not directly help anyone else who may need food. If you do not want to waste anything, simply put the leftovers in the refrigerator for a later time. And if that is not an option, decide whether the food left will be wasted on the plate or will be used as wasted energy in your body and stored as fat.

3.   Take a second piece on a take home plate if your friend or family member will be hurt if you do not have a second helping. Express your anticipation of enjoying it again at a later time.

4.   Remove yourself from the environment or from the people who pressure you before the situation even begins.

5.   Plan another event with your friend or family that does not center on food to help escape from "people pressure" to eat while still enjoying the company of the other person.

People pressure can certainly be intense and hard to deal with, but the most difficult detour remains.

The Detour of EMOTIONS

Special events, sights and smells, and people pressure may not cause you any detour delays. But, if you are feeling lonely or bored, upset or nervous, depressed or tense, or maybe even happy or relaxed, detours occur every time you turn the corner! Emotional triggers are not as easy to avoid because they can be unpredictable. It's a lot easier to avoid walking by the bakery at the grocery store than it is to control your feelings of boredom or depression. Is this detour inevitable? Probably, yes. Is it impossible to change your reactions to this detour? No!

Sometimes it seems that all of a sudden you find yourself halfway through the bag of chips before you even realize it. At first glance, it looks like you just went from feeling depressed to eating too much. But what may not be visible at first glance is *the chain of events* that occurred in between the "feeling" and the "consequence." For example, if you (1) have a bad day at work and are feeling depressed, (2) you find that you drive home (3) instead of going by the gym or (4) stopping to visit a friend. Once you walk through the front door, (5) you may not stop to change clothes or (6) read the mail but (7) walk directly into the kitchen. Once in the kitchen, (8) you may not take the time to look in the fruit bin to see what is there. (9) You open the pantry and (10) grab what is quickly available. You have a choice to open the bag, pull out a handful, close the bag, and return it to the pantry *before* you sit and eat your chips. However, (11) you take the bag with you, (12) sit on the couch, and (13) eat from the bag itself, without noticing how much has been eaten until you realize half the bag is empty. Thirteen links to the chain-all leading to one disastrous detour.

This is a *chain of events,* and with any chain, *it is only as strong as its weakest link.* Turn this scenario around, and look at what you can choose to do: (1) Knowing that you are depressed, (2) you decide to not even go home (3) until you go by the gym to walk, since exercise can help relieve depression. (4) Even if you do not feel like walking, you decide to at least avoid going home to a quiet house but (5) visit a friend (6) or go run some errands. (7) Once you arrive home, (8) you take time to change clothes before you enter the kitchen. (9) As you enter the kitchen, (10) you think about what you are really hungry for and (11) look for all the options available. (12) If you decide that you just HAVE to have chips, (13) you open the bag, and (14) remove your portion, then (15) return the bag back to the pantry. (16) You take your chips with you to the table, and (17) eat them slowly so that you do not miss even one bite of enjoyment from them! (18) Before you decide to get a second serving, you commit to remain where you are for about 15 minutes to allow your stomach time to realize that it has eaten. You may decide you still want more at this time, but at least you have taken steps to prevent a mindless response to an emotional detour. And you are much more aware of the effort required to go back for a second helping, which buys you more time to think through the consequences and whether you really are physically, or just emotionally, hungry.

It is obviously easier to avoid a major detour by breaking the chain early on in the sequence of events. The closer you are to the final turn into the detour, the harder it is to break the cycle of events; in other words, breaking the chain at #7 is easier than at #12, and breaking the chain at #3 is even better!

Look back at the times you know that you have eaten from an emotion and try to "put your car into reverse" and see the real chain of events that occurred. For example, were you too tired to go to the gym and exercise last week? Grabbed candy at work every time you passed the desk? Record the first behavior, or "chain link," and the last behavior, or "chain link," below:

First Chain Link (first behavior): _____

_____
_____
_____
_____

Last Chain Link (last behavior): _____

_____
_____
_____
_____

Spend some time thinking about that first and last behavior. What can you do differently between these two to break that emotional chain? Write different options to this scenario: _____

_____

_____

_____

Did you learn something about yourself in the process? You can break this chain by finding a way out of the detour--and the quicker you can change your pattern of behavior the easier it is to break its grip on you and your behaviors.

STRATEGY for DETOUR 4

To help you break an emotional chain of events, try these strategies:

1.   Stay alert to an emotional set-up. If you have had a bad day at work, expect that your emotions may try to convince you to take a detour. Awareness is over half of the battle!

2.   Keep your meals and snacks aligned in not only timing but also quality. Don't neglect that afternoon snack, and make sure you include protein fuel. This will ensure that any trigger to eat is not rooted in a physical craving from going too long between meals and snacks.

3.   Try to provide an alternative to eating as a way to feel better once you are aware of which emotions are triggers. What activities do you enjoy that relax or revive you? Do you like to listen to music? Do you enjoy going to a movie? Meeting a friend at the park for a walk? Taking a group exercise class? Enjoying a bubble bath or extra long shower? Think about an alternative that you can put in to action so that eating to feel better is not your only option.

4.   Keep a separate journal just for how you feel. Sometimes writing your thoughts on paper allows you to shorten the detour and control how you respond. Putting food in or writing it out-which choice will you make?

No matter what your triggers may be, every detour is a chance to learn more about yourself and how you handle bumps in the road. Each detour can make you stronger because you have a chance to learn how to keep control of your car as you face new, unexpected challenges.

A Look in the Rearview Mirror

Week 8: Dealing with Detours

Your **ACCELERATION Challenge** for Week 8: Note the specific detour that is most difficult for you. Review the strategies given for that detour and choose one to begin using this week. Write about your opportunities to use the new strategy in your Maintenance Log.

Now, record any changes you notice this week:

Date	Thoughts, Feelings, Body Changes?

The Rest of Your Life:

Your Maintenance Plan

"To this day, five years since starting Rev It Up!, I still try to eat every three to four hours and drink at least 64 ounces of water daily. More important to me, though, is the term I learned, 'more often than not.' It comes to play so many times for me. When I "fall off the wagon" and feel like I have failed myself by "cheating," I remember those words and that it is not the end of the world. I remember that I am still doing what is best for my health and my body 'more often than not' and that helps me to regain control again."   Rebecca

"As a result of Rev It Up!, I feel better, have lost weight and inches, and have a new outlook on food and eating."   Samuel

Chapter 22

Your Maintenance Plan

You did it! You have made it through 8 weeks of Rev It Up! challenges, and hopefully your body is feeling the benefits. Hard to believe, but it's now time to get serious about your long term maintenance plan. The newness of your healthy routines will wear off, just like the smell of a new car. But don't let your dedication begin to rust!

What do you do to keep your body's metabolism running smoothly and performing at its best? You perform routine checks to make sure everything is running smoothly-just like routine maintenance for your car. Doesn't sound exciting, but it is the key to a long life for a car; likewise, it is the key to a permanent lifestyle change for your body and your metabolism.

Where do you begin? First and most importantly, don't wait until you have a problem. Prevent a problem from happening in the first place by following the basic care guidelines from this Driver's Manual, your Rev It Up! principles:

1.   Listen to your body's hunger and fullness cues.
2.   Drink your daily eight cups of water, extra for exercise, and match up additional fluids.
3.   Align your meal and snack timing and content-plan ahead!
4.   Take time to do aerobic exercise and strength training each week--increase intensity for continued results.
5.   Follow the speed limits to eat at a reasonable pace.
6.   Tune up by choosing quality carbohydrate and fat fuel.
7.   Paint your car with 5 colors every day.
8.   Charge your battery by increasing exercise intensity periodically.
9.   Plan your pit stops carefully.
10. Clean your mirror to avoid distractions and stay focused.

11.   Prepare for detours with a strategic plan to get you back on track quickly.

12.   Evaluate your daily performance in your Maintenance Log.

You may be saying, "I know the list of things to do but how do I keep the momentum I have now? What maintenance plan can I follow to keep seeing results?" Think through the Four F's- FOUNDATION, FOOD, FLUID, and FITNESS. Which area has been the easiest for you? Which has been the most difficult? Some of the challenges are harder than others, but successful maintenance requires an action plan for all 4 areas. Don't neglect the challenges that are easy for you, but plan to spend more time on the areas where you encounter the most "potholes." The key to a maintenance plan that really works is: *think specific, be sure to think practical, and think small!* Many small victories lead to one big win!

Your FOUNDATION Goal and Maintenance Plan

Let's go through an example for each of the four F's, beginning with FOUNDATION. The Foundation challenges that you have faced include: 1) record hunger and fullness levels, 2) do not wait longer than 4 hours between meals and/or snacks, 3) experience a meal for 20 minutes and a snack for 10, 4) review your progress on a monthly basis and plan a reward for your efforts, 5) improve your body image by concentrating on positive traits and thoughts, and 6) increase awareness of the traps that create a detour for you (sights, sounds, smells; special events; people; emotions), and follow an escape plan to avoid them. So, for example, a FOUNDATION Goal such as "I'll eat more slowly at all meals" is good, but is not specific enough to help you take practical steps to make it a habit. A better strategy that's both practical and specific follows: "I will practice slowing down at dinner on three different days this week." The action steps are:

1.   Select Monday, Wednesday, and Friday dinner as practice meals.

2.   Highlight these days and meals on your calendar or day planner.

3.   Before beginning your meal, notice the clock.

4.   Eat, and linger, at the table until 20 minutes have passed.

5.   Answer these questions in your Maintenance Log during this time: "How full am I? Did this experience give less or more enjoyment?"

Now it's your turn:

My FOUNDATION Goal: _____

_____

_____

_____

The steps I will take (remember-think specific, practical, and small):

1.   _____

2.   _____

3.   _____

4.   _____

Your FOOD Goal and Maintenance Plan

One "F" down, three more to go! Let's move to FOOD. The FOOD challenges that you have faced include: 1) eating breakfast within 1 ½ hours of rising, 2) eating 3 to 4 fuel groups for a meal, 1 to 2 for a snack, and following portion guidelines, 3) eating five or more fruits and vegetables daily, 4) choosing high-quality carbohydrates like whole grains, 5) limiting your intake of saturated fats, fried foods, and high-fat condiments, and 6) choosing healthy selections when eating out. So, for example, a FOOD Goal such as "I'll eat more fruits and vegetables" is too broad and does not provide specific, real-life steps to measure your success. How will you know if you are really making progress in this area? "I'll eat more fruit each week" is a little better, but "I'll eat fruit for a morning snack on Monday through Thursday" is even better. Think *specific, practical, and small* when you think about your Maintenance Plan:

1.   Take a separate "produce run" every Sunday to purchase fresh fruits and vegetables for the week.
2.   Select fresh cut fruit and grapes for work snacks.
3.   Divide the fresh fruit into 4 individual containers on Sunday night.
4.   Bring one container to work on Monday through Thursday.
5.   Put a daily note by your keys to remind you to take your fruit snack.

Okay, it's your turn again!

My FOOD Goal: _____

_____

_____

_____

The steps I will take (specific, practical and small!):
1.   _____

_____

2._____

_____

3.   _____

_____

4.   _____

_____

Your FLUID Goal and Maintenance Plan

Is your Maintenance Plan making more sense now? Hopefully, yes! Now, take a moment to review your FLUID challenges, which include: 1) drink your daily eight cups of water, 2) drink extra for exercise, and 3) match up caffeine, artificially sweetened and alcoholic beverages with an equal amount of extra "match up" fluids (water, low-fat milk, tomato or vegetable juice). Now, for example, a FLUID Goal of "I'll drink more water" is too broad. But "I will drink 16 ounces of water as I drive to and from work Monday through Friday" is specific, practical, and small-step oriented. The action plan may look something like this:

1. Fill up your clean bottle with water the night before.
2. Put a note by your keys to remind you to take it with you when you drive.
3. Commit to drinking half of the water on the way to work.
4. If feasible, bring your water bottle inside and refrigerate.
5. Finish off your water bottle on the way home from work.
6. Wash and repeat!

Your turn, again!

My FLUID Goal: _____

_____

_____

_____

The steps I will take (you know the rules by now!):
1. _____

_____

2. _____

_____

3. _____

_____

4. _____

_____

Your FITNESS Goal and Maintenance Plan

The final F is often the most difficult: FITNESS! 1) Are you finding time to fit in four aerobic sessions a week, if weight loss is your goal? 2) Have you put pump power into action by doing two strength training sessions each week? 3) Do you make an effort to vary the intensity of your aerobic workouts on at least two of the four days? 4) Your strength training on at least one of the two days? Have you found a routine that works for you, either at home or in a local gym? If you stick with an exercise routine for about 20 weeks, or 5 months, it is very likely that you will exercise the rest of your life. But making fitness a priority in your weekly schedule can be so difficult.

Sometimes life just gets in the way, doesn't it? What obstacles have you encountered along the way?

One common obstacle involves **lack of commitment**. Do you feel that exercise gets shuffled to the bottom of your priority list once the day gets going? Too many demands which take too much of your time? Lack of commitment, for whatever reason, is a difficult bridge to cross. Or maybe your obstacle has been **lack of support**. Your desire to make new healthy habits may not be getting a lot of support from the home front. Maybe the problem is simply not having an exercise partner? If no one is expecting you at the gym, then no one will know if you don't show up, right? A third obstacle you may face is **lack of any variety**. The "same old, same old" gets boring, over time! And when your progress slows down, it's easy to be tempted to slow down your efforts, too. Last but not least, you may have just simply **lost your perspective** on *why* you exercise. The focus on health has been replaced with a focus on weight loss only. When the weight loss doesn't seem to match your efforts, do you feel depressed? Mad? Discouraged? Losing your focus narrows the path of success and can even block it completely. Ask yourself:

1.   Which of the four obstacles (lack of time, support, variety, or positive attitude) are you dealing with today?

_____

_____

2.   What type of activity, either aerobic or strength training, is most affected by this obstacle? _____

_____

Now that you have looked at which obstacle is your biggest challenge, create a new road map with a FITNESS Goal and Maintenance Plan. For example, your FITNESS goal could be "I will walk right after work on Tuesdays and Thursdays." List the small, practical steps that you will take to make this action plan work for you:

- Talk to your family about your new commitment.
- Write your workout appointment on your calendar for Tuesday and Thursday.

- Choose a route from your office, the gym, or your neighborhood.
- Change into your workout clothes BEFORE leaving work.
- Go to your planned location, and START WALKING!

My FITNESS Goal: _____

_____

_____

My Action Plan:

1. _____

2. _____

3. _____

4. _____

Have you realized yet that you have just completed your first *personalized* maintenance plan? You are now in charge of your continued progress, and you are *ready* and *able* to meet the challenges. As you work through this next week, remind yourself of just how far you have traveled. It is time to revisit Page 249 and take another Victory Lap! Record a list of the changes that you have seen in your body and in your relationship with food and exercise during the second month. And, of course, plan a reward-and give it to yourself-*this* week.

And finally...you can and should be proud of yourself. Even if you only managed to maintain one or two of the challenges, your metabolism is not the same today as it was when you started. Every small change makes a difference. If you have seen your body change an old habit (such as not drinking enough water) into a new healthier habit (drinking at least 8 cups of water daily), you have proven to yourself that your body is *capable* of change. The changes you have seen are a direct result of your hard work, and you can *own* these changes with confidence. Keep an eye on the road ahead, but don't miss the scenery that surrounds you-the accomplishments you and your body have made so far-as you enjoy the rest of the journey.

See you at the Finish Line!

What about the rest of your life?

Big question, isn't it? Rev It Up! is "a new way of living…a better way of feeling!" It is carefully designed to give you the steady encouragement and real-life guidelines that you need to actually own and maintain your new lifestyle. But being an owner means taking responsibility.

The principles for weight loss presented in Rev It Up! can be continued until you reach your desired weight range. Weight loss does not usually follow a steady, consistent pattern-you will experience ups and downs, and occasionally even hit a plateau that seems to linger longer than you'd like. When this happens, revisit the strategies presented throughout the program, especially Chapter 6, Balance Your Meals and Snacks, and Chapters 18 and 19, Charge Your Battery. Maybe your portions have gradually increased, or your body has adjusted to your exercise routines and needs a jump start to shake things up again. Read the "Most Frequently Asked Questions" section in the Appendix, especially Questions #1 through #4. These specifically deal with breaking weight plateaus and provide you simple strategies to get you back on track.

Once you have reached your goal range, you can experiment with fuel choices and portions-but depend on your hunger and fullness responses to those choices to help you make your decisions. Remember to relax-and enjoy the fact that you have reached your goal. Your body is not going to turn on you overnight and return back to where it started. Your metabolism is different, and your lifestyle proves that. What you do "more often than not" allows for occasional splurges-and your body is more capable of handling those splurges now. And take confidence that you will not want to return to your old habits, anyway.

Many, many individuals who lose weight, regardless of the specific program they follow, are successful in keeping it off-and you can be, too. Researchers have taken time to look at the common traits that these individuals have, regardless of what program they followed to lose the weight. In fact, the similarities between how they lost the weight are minimal (although diet and exercise changes are both required), but the similarities between how they are *keeping it off* are remarkably consistent. The keys are:

1. Keeping a daily journal for self assessment and monitoring.
2. Eating breakfast, consistently.
3. Having group support in place; family or friends that actively encourage them.
4. Regular physical activity, a consistent exercise program, and a commitment to simply live more actively-walk instead of drive, steps instead of elevators, etc.

These four habits are maintaining their weight loss, for the long haul. And you have these habits already in place, so the key is keeping them there!

Stay in touch. Go to the Web site, www.revitupfitness.com, and read Nutrition Tips that will help keep you on track. Become a friend on the Rev It Up! Fan page on Facebook, and chat with Tammy and other Rev It Up! alumni. Ask questions, share successes, and simply encourage each other on-line. Enjoy hearing from others who are revving it up…and enjoy *your* new way of living!

"It is amazing that total strangers are willing to reach out and help another total stranger get back on the pathway to healthier living. If I totally forgot everything I learned in Rev It Up! (which I haven't), just the support that I received in the last three days from other alumni of the program is worth every penny and then some! Due to the encouragement I received from just one person, I truly feel that I have made some headway this week and that definitely gives me the incentive to push on."   T.J.

Your Maintenance Log

Welcome to one of the most important parts of your journey-your Maintenance Log. Using these logs, you can quickly and clearly see areas in which you may need to work harder. But *more* importantly, you can see where you are succeeding, and what habits or patterns are changing for the better. It's a visible picture of how far you have come!

You will notice four goal boxes, one for each "F": Foundation, Food, Fluid, and Fitness. Use these boxes to highlight specific challenges on which you are working. These challenges are listed on the "Look in the Rearview Mirror" page at the end of each week. But you are not limited to these guidelines. Be as creative as you would like, and write down any helpful hints in your goal boxes that help you stay on track.

Set a goal to record *at least three days each week-two weekdays and one weekend day* (since we all know weekend eating can be very different from the rest of the week!). Follow these tips each time:

1. Record what and when you eat and drink, noting hunger (H) levels before you eat and fullness (F) levels after you eat.

2. Check off each cup of water you drink.

3. Write down any movement (aerobic activity) you complete, checking if you warm up, cool down, and stretch.

4. Write down any strength training you complete. Record the specific weight and number of repetitions for different exercises if desired. Watch your strength improve!

5. Take time to look back on your progress and compare notes. You may be amazed at how many changes you are making when you actually stop and look.

Consistent records reveal specific patterns unique to you and your lifestyle. So much can be learned with just five minutes of routine maintenance every day, so Rev It Up! and go for it!

Maintenance Log   S M T W T F S

Date: _____

Water

FOOD/BEVERAGE

H	Time	F
AM		
PM		

GOALS

Foundation

Food

Fluid

Fitness

AEROBIC

Activity: _____
Time: _____   HR: _____

Warm up ☐   Cool Down ☐   Stretch ☐

STRENGTH

Exercise	Lbs.	Rep Sets 1	2	3

Maintenance Log   S M T W T F S

Date: _____

Water

FOOD/BEVERAGE

GOALS

AEROBIC

Activity: _____
Time: _____   HR: _____

Warm up ☐   Cool Down ☐   Stretch ☐

STRENGTH

Exercise   Lbs.   Rep Sets
                        1   2   3

Foundation

Food

Fluid

Fitness

H | Time
AM

F

PM

Maintenance Log   S M T W T F S

Date: _____

Water

FOOD/BEVERAGE

H	Time
AM	
PM	

F

GOALS

Foundation

Food

Fluid

Fitness

AEROBIC

Activity: _____
Time: _____   HR: _____

Warm up ☐   Cool Down ☐   Stretch ☐

STRENGTH

Exercise	Lbs.	Rep Sets		
		1	2	3

Maintenance Log   S M T W T F S

Water _____

Date: _____

FOOD/BEVERAGE

H	Time	F
	AM	
	PM	

GOALS

Foundation

Food

Fluid

Fitness

AEROBIC

Activity: _____
Time: _____   HR: _____

Warm up ☐   Cool Down ☐   Stretch ☐

STRENGTH

Exercise	Lbs.	Rep Sets		
		1	2	3

Maintenance Log   S M T W T F S

Date: _____

Water

FOOD/BEVERAGE

H	Time	F
AM		
PM		

GOALS

Foundation

Food

Fluid

Fitness

AEROBIC

Activity: _____
Time: _____   HR: _____

Warm up ☐   Cool Down ☐   Stretch ☐

STRENGTH

Exercise	Lbs.	Rep Sets 1	2	3

Maintenance Log   S M T W T F S

Date: _____

Water _____

GOALS

Foundation

Food

Fluid

Fitness

AEROBIC

Activity: _____
Time: _____   HR: _____

Warm up ☐   Cool Down ☐   Stretch ☐

STRENGTH

Exercise   Lbs.   Rep Sets
                          1   2   3

FOOD/BEVERAGE

H | Time
F

AM

PM

Maintenance Log   S M T W T F S

Date: _____

Water

GOALS

Foundation

Food

Fluid

Fitness

FOOD/BEVERAGE

H	Time		F
AM			
PM			

AEROBIC

Activity: _____
Time: _____   HR: _____

Warm up ☐   Cool Down ☐   Stretch ☐

STRENGTH

Exercise	Lbs.	Rep Sets		
		1	2	3

Maintenance Log   S M T W T F S

Date:

Water

FOOD/BEVERAGE

H	Time	F
AM		
PM		

GOALS

Foundation

Food

Fluid

Fitness

AEROBIC

Activity: _____
Time: _____   HR: _____

Warm up ☐   Cool Down ☐   Stretch ☐

STRENGTH

Exercise	Lbs.	Rep Sets		
		1	2	3

Maintenance Log S M T W T F S

Date: _____

Water

FOOD/BEVERAGE

H	Time	F
	AM	
	PM	

GOALS

Foundation

Food

Fluid

Fitness

AEROBIC

Activity: _____
Time: _____   HR: _____

Warm up ☐   Cool Down ☐   Stretch ☐

STRENGTH

Exercise	Lbs.	Rep Sets		
		1	2	3

Maintenance Log   S M T W T F S

Date: _____

Water

FOOD/BEVERAGE

H | Time
AM

PM

F

GOALS

Foundation

Food

Fluid

Fitness

AEROBIC

Activity: _____
Time: _____   HR: _____

Warm up ☐   Cool Down ☐   Stretch ☐

STRENGTH

Exercise   Lbs.   Rep Sets
                        1   2   3

Maintenance Log S M T W T F S

Date: _____

Water

FOOD/BEVERAGE

H	Time	F
	AM	
	PM	

GOALS

Foundation

Food

Fluid

Fitness

AEROBIC

Activity: _____
Time: _____ HR: _____

Warm up [ ] Cool Down [ ] Stretch [ ]

STRENGTH

Exercise	Lbs.	Rep Sets		
		1	2	3

Maintenance Log   S M T W T F S

Date: _____

Water

FOOD/BEVERAGE

H	Time	F
	AM	
	PM	

GOALS

Foundation

Food

Fluid

Fitness

AEROBIC

Activity: _____
Time: _____   HR: _____

Warm up ☐   Cool Down ☐   Stretch ☐

STRENGTH

Exercise	Lbs.	Rep Sets		
		1	2	3

Maintenance Log   S M T W T F S

Date: _____

Water

FOOD/BEVERAGE

H	Time	F
AM		
PM		

GOALS

Foundation

Food

Fluid

Fitness

AEROBIC

Activity: _____
Time: _____   HR: _____

Warm up ☐   Cool Down ☐   Stretch ☐

STRENGTH

Exercise	Lbs.	Rep Sets		
		1	2	3

Maintenance Log   S M T W T F S

Date: _____

Water

FOOD/BEVERAGE

H	Time	F	
	AM		
	PM		

GOALS

Foundation

Food

Fluid

Fitness

AEROBIC

Activity: _____
Time: _____   HR: _____

Warm up ☐   Cool Down ☐   Stretch ☐

STRENGTH

Exercise	Lbs.	Rep Sets
		1 2 3

Maintenance Log   S M T W T F S

Date: _____

Water

FOOD/BEVERAGE

H | Time
AM

PM

F

GOALS

Foundation

Food

Fluid

Fitness

AEROBIC

Activity: _____
Time: _____   HR: _____

Warm up [ ]   Cool Down [ ]   Stretch [ ]

STRENGTH

Rep Sets

Exercise   Lbs.   1   2   3

Maintenance Log   S M T W T F S

Date: _____

Water

FOOD/BEVERAGE

H	Time	F
	AM	
	PM	

GOALS

Foundation

Food

Fluid

Fitness

AEROBIC

Activity: _____
Time: _____   HR: _____

Warm up ☐   Cool Down ☐   Stretch ☐

STRENGTH

Exercise	Lbs.	Rep	Sets 1 2 3

Maintenance Log　S M T W T F S

Date: _____

Water

FOOD/BEVERAGE

H	Time	F
AM		
PM		

GOALS

Foundation

Food

Fluid

Fitness

AEROBIC

Activity: _____
Time: _____　HR: _____

Warm up ☐　Cool Down ☐　Stretch ☐

STRENGTH

Exercise	Lbs.	Rep Sets		
		1	2	3

Maintenance Log　S M T W T F S

Date: _____

Water

GOALS

Foundation

Food

Fluid

Fitness

AEROBIC

Activity: _____

Time: _____　HR: _____

Warm up ☐　Cool Down ☐　Stretch ☐

STRENGTH

		Rep Sets		
Exercise	Lbs.	1	2	3

FOOD/BEVERAGE

H	Time	F
	AM	
	PM	

Maintenance Log   S M T W T F S

Date: _____

Water

FOOD/BEVERAGE

H	Time		F
	AM		
	PM		

GOALS

Foundation

Food

Fluid

Fitness

AEROBIC

Activity: _____
Time: _____   HR: _____

Warm up ☐   Cool Down ☐   Stretch ☐

STRENGTH

Exercise	Lbs.	Rep Sets		
		1	2	3

Maintenance Log   S M T W T F S

Date: _____

Water

FOOD/BEVERAGE

H	Time		F
AM			
PM			

GOALS

Foundation

Food

Fluid

Fitness

AEROBIC

Activity: _____
Time: _____   HR: _____

☐ Warm up   ☐ Cool Down   ☐ Stretch

STRENGTH

Exercise	Lbs.	Rep Sets		
		1	2	3

Maintenance Log S M T W T F S

Date: _____

Water

AEROBIC

Activity: _____
Time: _____ HR: _____

Warm up ☐ Cool Down ☐ Stretch ☐

STRENGTH

Exercise	Lbs.	Rep Sets		
		1	2	3

GOALS

Foundation

Food

Fluid

Fitness

FOOD/BEVERAGE

H	Time	F
	AM	
	PM	

Maintenance Log   S M T W T F S

Water

Date:

FOOD/BEVERAGE

H	Time	F
AM		
PM		

GOALS

Foundation

Food

Fluid

Fitness

AEROBIC

Activity: _____
Time: _____   HR: _____

Warm up ☐   Cool Down ☐   Stretch ☐

STRENGTH

Exercise	Lbs.	Rep Sets		
		1	2	3

Maintenance Log   S M T W T F S

Date: _____

Water

GOALS

FOOD/BEVERAGE

H	Time	F
	AM	
	PM	

Foundation

Food

Fluid

Fitness

AEROBIC

Activity: _____

Time: _____   HR: _____

Warm up ☐   Cool Down ☐   Stretch ☐

STRENGTH

Exercise	Lbs.	Rep Sets		
		1	2	3

Maintenance Log   S M T W T F S

Water

Date:

GOALS

Foundation

Food

Fluid

Fitness

FOOD/BEVERAGE

H | Time
AM

F

PM

AEROBIC

Activity: _____
Time: _____   HR: _____

Warm up ☐   Cool Down ☐   Stretch ☐

STRENGTH

Exercise   Lbs.   Rep Sets
                  1   2   3

Maintenance Log   S M T W T F S

Water

Date: _____

FOOD/BEVERAGE

H	Time	F
AM		
PM		

GOALS

Foundation

Food

Fluid

Fitness

AEROBIC

Activity: _____
Time: _____   HR: _____

Warm up ☐   Cool Down ☐   Stretch ☐

STRENGTH

Exercise	Lbs.	Rep Sets
		1 2 3

Maintenance Log   S M T W T F S

Water:

Date:

GOALS

AEROBIC

Activity: _____
Time: _____   HR: _____

☐ Warm up   ☐ Cool Down   ☐ Stretch

STRENGTH

Exercise	Lbs.	Rep Sets		
		1	2	3

Foundation

Food

Fluid

Fitness

FOOD/BEVERAGE

H	Time	F
	AM	
	PM	

Maintenance Log   S M T W T F S

Date: _____

Water

FOOD/BEVERAGE

H	Time	F
	AM	
	PM	

GOALS

Foundation

Food

Fluid

Fitness

AEROBIC

Activity: _____
Time: _____   HR: _____

Warm up ☐   Cool Down ☐   Stretch ☐

STRENGTH

Exercise	Lbs.	Rep Sets		
		1	2	3

Maintenance Log   S M T W T F S

Date:

Water

FOOD/BEVERAGE

H | Time

AM

PM

F

GOALS

Foundation

Food

Fluid

Fitness

AEROBIC

Activity: _____

Time: _____   HR: _____

Warm up ☐ Cool Down ☐ Stretch ☐

STRENGTH

Exercise   Lbs.   Rep Sets
                              1   2   3

Maintenance Log   S M T W T F S

Date:

Water

GOALS

AEROBIC

Activity: _____
Time: _____   HR: _____

Warm up [ ] Cool Down [ ] Stretch [ ]

STRENGTH

Exercise	Lbs.	Rep Sets		
		1	2	3

Foundation

Food

Fluid

Fitness

FOOD/BEVERAGE

H	Time	F
	AM	
	PM	

Maintenance Log   S M T W T F S

Water

Date: _____

FOOD/BEVERAGE

H	Time	F
AM		
PM		

GOALS

Foundation

Food

Fluid

Fitness

AEROBIC

Activity: _____
Time: _____   HR: _____

Warm up [ ]   Cool Down [ ]   Stretch [ ]

STRENGTH

Exercise	Lbs.	Rep Sets		
		1	2	3

Maintenance Log   S M T W T F S

Date: _____

Water

FOOD/BEVERAGE

H	Time	F
AM		
PM		

GOALS

Foundation

Food

Fluid

Fitness

AEROBIC

Activity: _____
Time: _____   HR: _____

Warm up ☐   Cool Down ☐   Stretch ☐

STRENGTH

Exercise	Lbs.	Rep Sets		
		1	2	3

Maintenance Log   S M T W T F S

Water

Date: _____

GOALS

AEROBIC

Activity: _____
Time: _____   HR: _____

☐ Warm up   ☐ Cool Down   ☐ Stretch

STRENGTH

Exercise	Lbs.	Rep Sets		
		1	2	3

Foundation

Food

Fluid

Fitness

FOOD/BEVERAGE

H	Time	F
AM		
PM		

Maintenance Log   S M T W T F S

Date: _____

Water

FOOD/BEVERAGE

GOALS

AEROBIC

Activity: _____
Time: _____   HR: _____

Warm up ☐   Cool Down ☐   Stretch ☐

STRENGTH

Exercise	Lbs.	Rep	Sets		
			1	2	3

Foundation

Food

Fluid

Fitness

H	Time		F
AM			
PM			

Victory Laps

What exactly is a victory lap? If you have ever seen a NASCAR driver celebrate after winning a big race, you know what a victory lap is! It's taking time to enjoy the moment, celebrate your win, and be proud of your accomplishments. It's as much a part of the race as the wave of the flag at the starting line!

The following table gives you an opportunity to record your own Rev It Up! victory laps. Each block represents a month. Write down the month in the left column, and list any and all of your victories during those four weeks. In the right column, plan and record how you are rewarding yourself. Repeat this exercise for each month, and enjoy celebrating your efforts. No one deserves it more!

My Victory Lap for the Month of _____	My Reward:

APPENDIX

Most Frequently Asked Questions

QUESTION #1: *I think I am "stuck"! I've lost weight, but now the scale is staying the same even though I don't think I'm doing anything different. What can I do to break this plateau?*

ANSWER: First of all, if you have a history of many attempts at weight loss, and have tried various programs with different measures of success, your body may be more resistance with each attempt. This is more common if your weight loss occurred too quickly. Your body's ability to lose weight may have slowed down, even if you can see positive changes in other ways, such as more energy and fewer cravings. Nevertheless, it is hard not to be frustrated about slow, or no, weight loss.

Secondly, over time, it is often easy to overestimate portions and/or amounts of added or hidden fats that creep into your daily foods. Since fats pack a lot of calories in a small amount, they can often be the contributor to slowed weight loss or a plateau. So try the following as your emergency plan to break your plateau and begin losing weight again: 1) Reduce your portion of grains (or "brown" carbohydrates) at the dinner meal by half. This is the meal that will most affect your weight since it is at the end of the day, when your body is slowing down naturally and burning fewer calories in preparation for bedtime. Or you can decide to completely eliminate grains at the dinner meal only for a temporary period of time, but don't neglect to follow the next step. 2) Make up the difference in carbohydrate energy by substituting more color (more vegetables) at this same dinner meal. Double up on those veggies! 3) Eliminate fats "more often than not," meaning, NO added ping pong ball of fats or fried foods or cream sauces on four to five days out of the week. This is a more extreme step, but can save you quite a bit of unknown calories. Limiting added fats to only two or so days a week allows you to get in the healthy fats (the unsaturated fat choices) that you need for the essential fatty acids and fat soluble vitamins but reduces the possibility of getting too many extra calories from fats on a daily basis. 4) Maintain your water intake, and 5) Keep striving for four sessions of cardio activity each week, with two of the four sessions incorporating strength training as well. Most importantly, do *not* give up!

QUESTION #2: *I have been so stressed at work, and for some reason it makes me feel like eating all the time. My meal timing is off, and I just can't seem to get back on track. I found myself eating my third brownie yesterday even though I wasn't hungry, and now I feel so guilty! What's wrong with me?*

ANSWER: Stress is a very real situation in which we all find ourselves from time to time. So what exactly does stress do to your body, besides make your heartbeat faster, blood pressure rise, mood turn irritable and interfere with a good night's sleep? Stress actually uses or burns more energy (calories), especially the type of energy that supplies a chemical called serotonin. This chemical is produced by carbohydrates, so this helps explain why you tend to eat more when you are stressed and often want quick carbohydrates like sugars.

As stress burns energy, it simultaneously triggers the release of adrenaline and cortisol, two hormones called the "flight or fight" hormones-which help in emergencies-but may not be much help when you are at work, trying to meet a deadline, and have nowhere to run *or* no one to fight! The natural tendency is to eat carbohydrates, which trigger your brain to produce serotonin, a chemical that relaxes and calms you. This calming effect can be produced by a handful of whole wheat crackers, but often a handful of cookies are more appealing.

First of all, declare your desk, your computer, your television, loud music and any other distractions off limits until *after* you eat something. Try to plan ahead for these inevitable moments by keeping an "emergency snack pack" available. Avoid higher sugar, simple carbohydrate foods as much as possible, which can actually *increase* your appetite even more. Choose whole grains and a little lean protein such as a mozzarella cheese stick and whole-wheat crackers, or peanut butter and apple slices. Not convenient to have that kind of snack available? Prepare ahead by having your own trail mix of whole-wheat cereal squares mixed with slivered almonds and raisins handy, or have an energy bar made with protein and complex carbohydrates.

No matter what, slow down and give yourself a 10-minute break to fuel your brain with *good* fuel, relax those stress hormones and boost your energy. And if emotions sometimes take over and you dive into a plate of brownies, try to clear your head by sitting down, taking it slow, savoring every bite and adding a little protein-like a cold glass of milk-to diffuse that quick rush and fall. Mainly, get right back on track and don't let guilt cloud your way. Remember, it is what you do *more often than not* that guides your body's metabolism rate!

QUESTION #3: *I have really gotten off track, and blown it way too many times. I feel like giving up. What should I do?*

ANSWER: Don't let occasional splurges get you off track! Remember, "one lapse does NOT a relapse make"! Keep in mind the following tips as you continue taking small steps forward: 1) *Do not focus on calories-focus only on fuel groups!* Had a few doughnuts for breakfast, and wishing you hadn't? Don't skip lunch to make up the calories. Instead, try to round out what was missing at breakfast. Look for lean proteins, veggies, and low-fat dairy for lunch. That would be a great time to have a grilled chicken salad with lots of greens, vegetables and some grated cheese, with low-fat dressing on the side so you control the amount. Having a hard time getting those colors into your meals? Double up at one meal, like extra lettuce and bell pepper slices in your pita sandwich (You can ask for extra even at a fast food sandwich place!) Think balance, and think fuel groups, and just catch up on the missing pieces at the next meal. 2) *Do a quick review of what you ate at the last meal and/or snack.* Remembering what you have eaten most recently may help encourage you to eat less the next time around. Remember, "I CAN EAT AGAIN…just not right now!", and 3) *Never be fooled into skipping the next meal to punish yourself for a splurge.* Missing an entire meal to make up for too many calories at the previous will *always* backfire on you.

The key is balancing your fuel groups, trusting your hunger, and learning from your lapses. Failure is not possible. How can something be a failure when you can learn so much about yourself? The biggest splurge can result in more self awareness of the "why" behind your choice, which can result in greater confidence and motivation for the next time you find yourself in the same situation.

Eating better starts with just one meal--one day--one week at a time. Unhealthy patterns do not happen over night but over a long period of days that lead to weeks that lead to months that lead to years. Likewise, healthy patterns take time, so be patient. It's worth it!

QUESTION #4: *Why does the scale seem to fluctuate so much? I can gain 2 or 3 pounds overnight, even if I haven't done anything to justify it! What causes that?*

ANSWER: You have discovered how fickle the scales can be. They never really tell the whole story. Did you know that an overcast or stormy day can actually add several pounds to the scale? Low pressure keeps water in your tissues, and since our bodies are mostly water, an overcast day can make us "gain weight"…that is, fluid! Did you know (well, at least most women do!) that hormones can add 2 to 6 pounds over a three to seven day length of time? Anti-inflammatory drugs, like ibuprofen, or steroid type drugs for allergies may cause temporary fluid retention, resulting in temporary weight gain. Even not getting enough sleep may slow down your body's ability to burn carbohydrates, which makes more glucose available for fat storage, and increases the stress hormone cortisol, which stimulates your appetite for rich, high-fat foods. And did you realize that just three shakes of salt, or ½ teaspoon, can add 1 pound of body weight? One gram of sodium can hold onto 16 ounces of water, and that equals a pound. So that dinner at the local Japanese restaurant may explain why your clothes fit tighter the next day-salt!

So try not to obsess about the pounds on that scale. Remind yourself that your body's weight is a combination of water, muscle, bone, fat, and body tissues…so any change on that scale is *not* just a reflection of fat alone. About 65% of our body weight comes from water, so most quick body weight fluctuations are a result of water changes only. Don't get on the scale more often than once a week. Keep following the Rev It Up! principles, and enjoy how your body feels, the increasing self-confidence you are gaining, the changes you see in your strength and aerobic ability, the way your clothes fit, and the power that comes from taking charge of your wellness and health. Don't let a single number take that away from you.

QUESTION #5: *How do I tell if something is "whole grain"? What's the difference in whole-wheat or whole grain, anyway?*

ANSWER: Whole-wheat is always the same as whole grain, but not all whole grains are whole-wheat. Confused even more? That simply means that whole grain can mean whole-wheat OR whole grain corn or whole grain rice (brown rice), or any combination of the grains out there. So any bread that is listed as a multi-grain bread, like 7 grain, would be a great choice. And any bread listed as 100% whole-wheat or whole-wheat bread is a great choice. Don't be fooled by the label "wheat bread" alone, though, since that is really just brown-colored white bread. Regardless, even if white bread or white rice breaks down much more quickly than whole grain foods, if you eat these "white" foods with some kind of protein, the process slows down and does not produce a quick "rush" of carbohydrate calories. So when you can, choose whole grain, but when you cannot, you can still eat the lower fiber grain-just make sure you add protein to that meal or snack to help balance your body's response.

QUESTION #6: *I am heading to the beach with my family for summer break and am worried about what I am going to eat. I just love this seafood buffet at my favorite restaurant there. Do I have to avoid it completely?*

ANSWER: Summer vacation eating-how can you handle all of those temptations available? Try these suggestions: 1) Budget your fats. If you know you want to order fried shrimp, strip the fat from your breakfast and lunch meals so you have room for extra fats in the evening, 2) Balance a dessert by choosing a low-fat main course and lots of color (vegetables and/or fruits) as your side dishes instead of pastas, rice or potato. Plan to share it with someone else to save a few calories without missing out! 3) Beware of "drinking" all of your calories. A pina colada or strawberry daiquiri (7 ounces) can contain over 500 calories and over 17 grams of fat. Drinks that are mixed with cream, milk, fruit juice or soda can pack more calories, so remember to take that into account when ordering, and 4) Plan an after-meal activity, such as a beach volleyball game after breakfast, or skiing after lunch, or a sunset walk after dinner. This not only will burn calories but also help you limit heavier food choices at the meal knowing you are going to be active afterwards.

QUESTION #7:   *My friend told me that I need to exercise every day, but I don't have time to go to the gym 7 days a week. How can I burn more calories outside of the gym?*

ANSWER: Aerobic exercise and strength training are very important for weight loss and maintenance. However, you can burn extra calories every single day by adding just a few small movements or changing a few simple behaviors. Try these: 1) Use "standing in line" at the grocery store or gas station as a chance to flex your abs or tighten your rear end (no one will know, honest!). It's like having your own "butts and guts" conditioning class on a mini scale! 2) Do calf raises while talking on the telephone. 3) If you have stairs at home, take them *each* time you do a load of laundry instead of accumulating all the loads into one before you make the trip. 4) Do crunches or push ups while watching TV-maybe not every time, but occasionally? 5) If you really want to make your family think you have lost it, do jumping jacks during commercials. Your younger kids will think this is a great new game (and your teenager already expects odd behavior from you anyway!), and 6) Do stretches in the shower, like neck rolls and shoulder shrugs. Remember, it's what you do more often than not that counts. Wellness is a lifestyle-not just an aerobics class. Enjoy your day, and get *moving*!

QUESTION #8:   *I've been invited to a holiday party this weekend. Any tips on how to handle all those temptations?*

ANSWER: Here are a few health tips to take with you when you go: 1) Do not arrive at the big event hungry! Make sure you eat breakfast, lunch, and an afternoon snack as usual, because saving your day's calories for one big meal does not work! However, feel free to lighten up the fat content at those earlier meals. 2) Survey the entire table *before* you start filling your plate. Choose two or three items that are worth every bite, and skip the other higher-fat party choices like chips and dip that you can have anytime. 3) Enjoy your choices, but keep those portions small. You can have more items if you have smaller portions of each. 4) Wait about 20-30 minutes after eating before going back for seconds. Ask yourself, "Am I really physically hungry for more?", and 5) Drink a glass of water between every serving of alcohol or sweetened beverage. This will not only decrease calories but also slow the appetite-stimulating effect of alcohol and/or sugars.

QUESTION #9: *I hate to write in my journal. Do I have to?*

ANSWER: Journaling is the best way to visualize your progress. And it is one of the top three habits of people who have lost weight and kept it off over time. But it can be a hassle, especially when your lifestyle is fast paced and your schedule is full. Start simply by choosing small steps, like picking three days out of seven and journal those completely. Or if that is too much to assume, then at least journal the meal(s) that is most difficult for you. Dinner? Lunch? Afternoon snack? The journals are for *you*-to spend time with yourself (how often do we really do that?) and to get to know what triggers overeating for you, to understand when your biggest food challenges hit –and to see your progress. Don't forget that important point of journaling! How else are you going to be able to really see and applaud the changes that you are making unless they are written down?

QUESTION #10: *I don't really want to lose weight, I just want to learn to eat better and live a healthier lifestyle. Can I follow Rev It Up! anyway?*

ANSWER: Certainly! You will probably need to adjust your portion guidelines higher-but keeping an eye on your hunger and fullness will help you quickly discover if you are fueling for four hours, or over- or under-doing it! You learn by trial and error, and adjustments can be made, up or down, as needed for you. Rev It Up! is a healthy way of living for all bodies and ages and allows the flexibility you need to meet your energy goals, even if weight loss is not necessary.

QUESTION #11: *Is bottled water better for me than tap water?*

ANSWER: Not necessarily. Bottled water is everywhere, and sales of more than 2 billion a year certainly indicate it's here to stay. You may buy it just because it tastes better or you may be concerned about the safety of your own tap water. But as a general rule, you do not have to drink bottled water to stay safe.

By law, public water sources must be regularly monitored and tested for contamination. One of the more serious concerns has been the question of lead in public drinking water. You can have your tap water tested if you are worried, and a call to the Environmental Protection Agency Safe Drinking Water Hotline (1-800-426-4791) can direct your steps. But an easy way to decrease the amount of lead in your tap water is to "flush it out." Simply run the water through the faucet until it becomes as cold as possible. This helps for two reasons: First, it guarantees that water you end up drinking has not been exposed over a long period of time to pipes containing lead. Secondly, colder water is less susceptible to "grabbing and holding on" to the lead from the pipe itself.

Did you know that 25% of bottled waters are actually tap water that has been packaged to sell? A company is free to use water from a public source and bottle it in plastic containers for a profit. High-end brands, such as Perrier or Evian, are certainly not tap water, but your local or less-expensive versions may be. Regardless, most bottled water companies are members of the International Bottled Water Association, which ensures that they follow careful standards and are inspected yearly. One current concern to consider, especially if you have young children in your home, is that most bottled waters do not supply the right amount of fluoride to prevent cavities. However, bottled water companies are looking at this issue and several companies fortify their water with fluoride already.

So, bottled water or tap water? It's your choice. Consider your
pocketbook, your home source of tap water, and your motivation to
drink water in the first place. Find your favorite source, and commit
to drink it daily.

QUESTION #12: *What about vitamins? Do I need to take a daily
supplement?*

ANSWER: It depends on the individual. If you eat whole grains,
lean meats, low-fat dairy, and lots of fruits and vegetables, the
answer is "not really." But the reality is-you probably don't, at least
not yet, until you complete the eight weeks of Rev It Up! Therefore,
you may want to consider taking a multivitamin/mineral supplement
that provides 100% of the RDA, or recommended daily allowances,
of the nutrients you need for your age and gender. Do you need to
spend a lot of money on specialized natural vitamins, or can you buy
an over-the-counter version at your supermarket?   The choice is
yours, but the more expensive, natural vitamins are not necessary for
most people. Regardless of the type, look for the USP label to ensure
that it meets official standards for dietary supplements (www.usp-
dsvp.org). In regards to specific minerals like calcium, do you need
to take an additional supplement? Yes, if you do not consume three
dairy servings every day. A daily multivitamin/mineral supplement
does not provide over 10-15% of the recommended levels of
calcium, usually. There is simply not enough room to include all that
you need! An additional calcium supplement from a carbonate or
citrate source is preferred, and usually comes in 500-600 mg tablets.
An adult female should consume 1200 mg/day; therefore, one to two
tablets   in   addition   to   your   multivitamin   supplement   are
recommended (depending on how much dairy you consume). Do
make sure that your calcium supplement contains Vitamin D. Recent
research indicates that Americans need more Vitamin D than
originally thought to ensure optimal bone health.

QUESTION #13: *How do I choose the right energy bar for a
snack? There are too many options, and I'm confused!*

ANSWER: Energy bars can be a convenient snack that meets the "two fuel group" requirement but not all bars are worth the effort or money.   Since a variety of products are available, ask the following questions:

1.   Does the product have a nutrition fact label? (If not, avoid it!)
2.   Does the product sound too good to be true? (It probably is!)
3.   What does the product claim to do? Does research back it up?

Once you have answered these questions, follow these guidelines to make the best choice for you:

1.   Choose a bar that is equal to a snack – not a meal! These foods are "engineered" and do not contain the same amount of fiber and nutrients found naturally in foods.
2.   Read the label. Look for an average of 200 calories, 10+ grams of protein, < 8 grams of added fats, primarily unsaturated, and preferably 3+ grams of fiber.
3.   Higher protein bars can fit in certain circumstances, but be aware that they are usually more expensive, often taste chalky and unpalatable, and require extra fluid intake.
4.   Avoid herbal additives if taking prescription medications because many can interact adversely.
5.   Read the labels carefully! DO NOT USE PRODUCTS CONTAINIING EPHEDRINE, MA HUANG, YOHIMBE AND/OR MATE.

QUESTION #14: *Are there any free Web sites that you recommend that provide nutrition or fitness information?*

ANSWER: Yes! The following list is not comprehensive, but provides you with a variety of Web sites for nutrition and fitness information. These are free to online users, but some may require registration.

1. www.eatright.org (the Web site for the American Dietetic Association)
2. www.fitday.com (an online tool for calculating calories consumed and burned every day)
3. www.sparkpeople.com (another online tool for calculating calories consumed every day)
4. www.myrecipes.com (the Web site for all Oxmoor House publications, such as Cooking Light, Health, and Southern Living magazines. Look for the Rev It Up! weight management tips coming in January 2010!)
5. www.healthierus.gov/dietaryguidelines (the Web site for the U.S. Department of Health and Human Services. New 2010 Dietary Guidelines coming soon)
6. www.webmd.com (an online tool that provides health information for the entire family)
7. www.healthydiningfinder.com (an online tool that highlights healthy menu items for fast food and sit-down restaurants that have been approved by registered dietitians)

Note: the inclusion of these Web site addresses does not constitute an endorsement of any one site. At the time of publication, all Web sites were operable.

Sample One-Day Menu Ideas
Using Rev It Up! Guidelines

Example 1: Energy provided by grains, fruits and vegetables	Example 2: Energy provided by fruits and vegetables only
BREAKFAST: Whole grain English muffin Scrambled egg w/ 2% cheese (1 egg and 1 ppb cheese) Cantaloupe, 1 bb	**BREAKFAST:** Egg omelet w/ 2% cheese, tomato and green pepper (2 eggs and 1 ppb cheese) Cantaloupe, 1 bb 1% milk, 1 cup
SNACK: Nectarine, 1 bb	**SNACK:** Nectarine, 1 bb
LUNCH: Whole-wheat tortilla wrap, 1 bb Sliced turkey breast, palm size Lettuce shreds, diced tomato Fresh fruit cup, 1 bb 1% milk, 1 cup	**LUNCH:** Sliced turkey breast, palm size 2% cheese, 1 ppb Blend of lettuces, grape tomatoes, cucumbers Raspberry vinaigrette, 1 ppb 1% milk, 1 cup
MID-AFTERNOON SNACK: Lemon low-fat yogurt, 1 bb Frozen or fresh blueberries, 1 bb	**MID-AFTERNOON SNACK:** Apple slices, 1 bb Peanut butter, 1 ppb
DINNER: Grilled salmon, palm size Brown rice w/ mushrooms, 1 bb Broccoli, carrot mix, 1 bb Mixed greens salad Balsamic vinaigrette, 1 ppb	**DINNER:** Grilled salmon, palm size Grilled vegetables: zucchini, squash and carrot chunks Mixed greens salad Balsamic vinaigrette, 1 ppb
1 bb = 1 baseball	**1 ppb = 1 ping pong ball**

These two examples are based on weight-loss guidelines for an average female. Both days are approximately the same calorie level, but offer two alternatives for energy sources. Example 1 is designed using whole grains, fruits and vegetables, with animal, plant, and dairy proteins; Example 2 is designed using *only* fruits and vegetables, with animal, plant, and dairy proteins. Both provide energy and protein, but allow you the freedom to choose energy sources.

My Personal Rev It Up! Journey

Tammy Beasley, RD, CSSD, LD
Author and Creator, Rev It Up!

If you are reading this now, you have made a decision to commit, or are considering a commitment, to learn and live the Rev It Up! lifestyle. First of all, thank you for the trust you have placed in me and this program. I know that countless programs are available, and an endless stream of information bombards you daily from magazines, radio, and television. Because of this, I feel it is important to give you an opportunity to look inside the window into how Rev It Up! came to be in the first place. Where did the ideas come from? On what are the principles based? How is it different from all the other programs out there? Is it worth your time and financial commitment? Can you trust what you learn and are asked to practice? Will it make a difference in your life? Because of all of these questions, and more, I would like to share the story of my own personal Rev It Up! journey.

In 1984, I graduated from Auburn University with a degree in nutrition and foods, and headed to the University of Alabama in Birmingham to complete my dietetic internship. My decision to major in nutrition was not the first path I took when entering Auburn. Born in Huntsville, Alabama, the Rocket City and home of NASA and the Marshall Space Flight Center, an engineering path was encouraged and expected. I gave it a two year effort but I quickly discovered that even if my brain could make the grades, my heart was not in it. More importantly, the stress of those first years in combination with a compulsive, perfectionist personality led to my first experience with an eating disorder. My 5'6" frame dropped to 106 pounds, and it took a concerned family and a wise physician to make me recognize that the increasing stress I felt, decreasing grades I received, frequent illnesses I had, and overall anxiety I experienced were a result of poor nutrition. Realizing that my nutritional health had affected every part of my life, I was compelled to find out more about this field that combined science, psychology, and human behavior-a field that influenced every person, in every family, including my own. And I loved it!

The year in graduate school at UAB provided me a wide range of clinical experiences, where I saw firsthand how nutrition affects healing, wellness, and even psychological health. I was especially challenged by the nutrition support rotations, involving critically ill patients on total parenteral nutrition-where the nutritional medicine entering their veins could make a difference in life or death. Rotations in weight management, eating disorders, and even sports nutrition were not available outside of the occasional outpatient clinics. It didn't really matter to me, though. Surely my clinical experience and expertise should not be "wasted" on simple weight loss issues but used on more "important" causes, like renal disease or cancer treatment, right?! So I thought as I joined the UAB staff as a clinical dietitian for the gastrointestinal medicine unit.

It did not take long, however, before I realized that issues of weight management and how a person feels about body image infiltrated the care of almost every patient with whom I worked. And whether you could say I was in the right place at the wrong time, or the wrong place at the right time, after barely a year in practice, I was given the responsibility to create a weight-loss program for patients who would be undergoing the "gastric bubble procedure." The gastric bubble program included insertion of a balloon-type device in the stomach that would not allow as much food to be consumed and digested; therefore, these obese patients would be forced to eat less and as a result, lose weight. Of course, the weight loss would be permanent, if they simply followed the rules. As I worked with each client, I realized that my three or four visits and folder full of handouts hardly made a dent in changing life-long eating habits and mindsets.

These patients were in trouble, and I felt great responsibility to make a lasting difference, and great frustration when I saw few changes embraced. What was I doing wrong? What could I do differently, and what could the patient do differently? Why did the most motivated patient also struggle with consistent weight loss-even when following all the rules I gave him or her? The medical team found out that the gastric bubble did NOT work, and the procedure was no longer allowed. And I found out that weight loss was a lot more complicated and serious than I had perceived-even if all the knowledge was available.

My clinical interests began to change, and, yet again, I found myself in a situation where I was asked to direct another controversial weight loss program. This time, it was a fasting program, following on the heels of the popularity of the Optifast diet. UAB wanted to be on the cutting edge and was planning to offer a fasting program to the public, but I could not bring myself to commit to the idea that 400 calories, of liquids only, would produce anything other than quick weight loss and long-term problems with weight maintenance as well as health complications. So I studied, and researched, and created a new program that would solve the problem of quick weight regain-UAB would *double* the calories in its program and provide 800 instead! We would add behavioral modification sessions, and support from full time psychologists. Our program would make a difference, and I was proud to be on the cutting edge.

But guess what? Yet again, many patients had great success, if you look at success as weight loss only. Many patients attended every behavioral class, every nutrition class, and followed all the rules – but most of the patients failed to keep the majority of their weight off once the fasting portion ended. I will never forget how confused and discouraged and broken-hearted I felt when my favorite, most compliant patient called in tears, unable to prevent weight regain no matter what advice I gave and she followed. What had happened to these patients' metabolisms during these weeks and months? Had I contributed to a damaging cycle that would only worsen for them?

As I struggled with these questions, I was offering sports nutrition counseling after hours at a local fitness center through another hospital. Athletes would make an appointment to discuss how they could lower their body fat, eat for more energy, and improve performance in competitions. The atmosphere was quite opposite of what I saw in the hospital clinic. For the most part, these were health-oriented clients who only wanted the facts-none of that "touchy feeling" stuff. They were driven to perform, and wanted to know grams of carbohydrates and fats and proteins and how it affected their next race or workout. I enjoyed this arena, but was unaware of how it was affecting me personally. Sometimes an athlete would go overboard in his or her compulsiveness, and I began noticing some disordered eating behaviors over time. At the same time, I watched the obese clients from the clinic struggle with their own version of disordered eating. And I began pushing myself harder-since I had to be an example to others, I had to be one step ahead...one pound thinner...one minute faster...or I would lose credibility.

The more I pushed myself, the more panicked I would get and the more secret my eating behaviors became. Until I was into another eating disorder trap-this time, the compulsive overeating of fat-free ("good for you") foods, and the subsequent guilt from my lack of willpower, and the resulting drive to exercise even more and try to eat even less. It never worked more than a few days...I'd be back at square one. Able to encourage my clients to be kind to their bodies and take changes gradually, I was unable to give myself any comfort, grace, or acceptance.

Although I did not realize it at the time, my actions and words were a silent cry for help. My co-worker and friend, a psychologist by trade, confronted my behaviors-and I was finally able to see my behaviors for what they really were. The journey out of that circle was not easy, and involved taking a harder look inside at what was behind my behaviors and a softer look outside at what was realistic and healthy. I had been taught the fat grams, cholesterol content, fiber sources, calorie count for *every* food and drink. My brain was a walking calorie computer, ready to convert fat grams to percent calories with every bite. I had to learn to *shut the calorie calculator off*, for good, and learn to eat from hunger and stop eating when full. Learn to eat balanced, and include all foods in moderation. And what freedom it was!!! I will never forget eating pizza again after three years of missing out. It had never tasted quite so good, because it represented a freedom that I had not allowed myself for too long.

And the interesting thing is-as my mind became more balanced, my weight became steady and consistent, my eating became more balanced and calm, and my life became more full and rich. Self esteem struggles? Sure, I still have them sometimes, but I do not reach for another barbell or eat another cookie or rice cake, for that matter, to make it go away. The self-punishment behaviors do not automatically follow. In fact, they don't exist at all anymore! I have to work through my thoughts and emotions, and it's not always fun, but I find that I am back to more self acceptance within a few hours, or maybe a day or two, depending. Self-punishment by exercising and eating, or not, is long gone. And that "loss" is my greatest gain!

This three-year process of personal recovery concluded with meeting my husband-to-be, and marrying him within six months later. That marriage, however, meant a move to Miami, Florida, where for the next nine years, I lived in a world that literally breeds eating disorders and body image distortions. From the safety net of Alabama to the cross-cultural tangle of Miami, I had to grow up quickly. Professionally, I was not sure what direction I would take, and not being bilingual actually hindered me from receiving employment for the first year. However, a local hospital was interested in developing an outpatient nutrition counseling program, and I was hired to do just that. Within the first month, a hospital physician asked if I had ever counseled clients with eating disorders. This led to long discussions and the opportunity to begin working with an incredible professional team of psychologists, psychiatrists, and physicians specializing in this field.

At first I was concerned that my own personal history would be a hindrance, but I quickly discovered a great passion for this area of nutrition. My own experiences proved helpful and insightful and often opened a door for deeper trust between myself and my client. I pursued an additional certification as an eating disorder specialist in nutrition through the International Association of Eating Disorder Professionals (IAEDP), which I completed in 1993 and continue to maintain today. So my professional years in Miami concentrated on working with women and men, of all ages, who struggled with some type of disordered eating-the young grade school student, the high school athlete, the college undergraduate, the business professional, the at-home mom, and the list goes on.

Each client taught me something unique, and the medical team with which I worked provided tremendous support for personal and professional growth. I am so thankful for those years! However, after the birth of my two sons, my husband and I had the opportunity to move back home, to Alabama where my family lives and near the Tennessee state line, where his family lives. We took the chance, and I took a year off to help myself and my children adjust to what I now know as "reverse culture shock." I know I grew up physically here in Huntsville, but I grew up emotionally and professionally in Miami. It took some time to feel comfortable again in a city where the majority of people speak English-and Southern style at that!

After a year, I became a part time nutrition consultant for a local fitness center, and continued to see not only athletes but also clients with disordered eating. As time progressed, I heard myself continually teaching each client about his or her body, how it really works, and what it does to try to *help,* which often ends up only hurting. I heard myself encouraging behavior changes in the same way to each client, whether he was a competitive cyclist wanting to improve his time, she was a businesswoman trying to manage signs of early diabetes, or he or she was a young student struggling with body image. The athlete needed to learn how to listen to his own body's hunger and fullness cues and benefited from more attention given to the "why" instead of just the "what." The client with an eating disorder needed to know what foods would provide the most energy and when a meal or snack should be eaten and benefited from this practical knowledge. The inside look at "why" with an outside look at "what" and "when" proved to be powerful tools for change for *both* types of clients.

So, in December of 2000, I sat down and began writing a manual that I hoped would combine all I had learned in my professional and personal journey towards eating and living well. I wanted to translate onto paper the information that I shared in consultation after consultation, and thus, Rev It Up! was born! My initial class knew they were my "trial group" and had little more than a folder of handouts from which to work. But the privilege of watching lifestyle changes take place, and hope in their bodies restored where little was left, continued to motivate me to make Rev It Up! even more user-friendly, practical and whole. I began to offer the teaching tools I used to other registered dietitians, and to date, Rev It Up! has been taught in 25 states through the United States by over 55 registered dietitians. Each class, each person, has contributed in some way to this book as it reads today. Rev It Up! is a program that initiates one change at a time, creating a different way of thinking about the body and its relationship with food and exercise. A program that encourages each participant to *own* the changes he or she creates and maintains. A program that offers a new way of living and a better way of feeling about yourself and your body.

Is Rev It Up! the only answer for America's struggle with weight, for *your* struggle with your own body? Of course not-many wonderful programs are available-but I believe, without a doubt, that it offers a simple way to break through the barriers that can prevent long term weight loss and a powerful, new way of thinking about yourself and your body's potential.   Again, thank you for your commitment to and trust in the program, and may your Rev It Up! journey lead you to a healthier lifestyle, a more confident mindset, and a life well-lived!

References

Rev It Up! is the result of over 25 years of experience as a registered, licensed dietitian-experience that includes a variety of clinical rotations, five directorships of weight-management programs, three contracts as a sports nutrition consultant to a fitness facility or wellness center, over 15 years of specialization in the field of eating disorders, and, most importantly, hundreds and hundreds of individual nutrition consultations. Specific references for each chapter of Rev It Up! would be impossible to list; however, the following includes the professional references that have been most influential on my practice over the years.

Clark, N (1990, 1997). Nancy Clark's Sports Nutrition Guidebook (2nd edition). Champaign, IL: Human Kinetics.

Kleiner, S.M. (1998). Power Eating: Build Muscle, Gain Energy, Lose Fat. Champaign, IL: Human Kinetics.

McArdle, W.D., Katch, F.I., and Katch, V.L. (1991). Exercise Physiology: Energy, Nutrition and Human Performance. Malvern, PA: Lea & Febiger.

McKardle, W.D., Katch, F.I., and Katch, V.L. (1999) Sports and Exercise Nutrition. Baltimore, MD: Lippincott Williams & Wilkins.

Reiff, D.W. and Reiff, K.K. (1992). Eating Disorders: Nutrition Therapy in the Recovery Process. Gaithersburg, MD: Aspen Publishers, Inc.

Rodin, J. (1992). Body Traps. New York: William Morrow and Company, Inc.

Vredevelt, P., Newman, D., Beverly, H., and Minirth, F. (1992). The Thin Disguise: Overcoming and Understanding Anorexia and Bulimia. Nashville, TN: Thomas Nelson Publishers.

Zerbe, K.J. (1993). The Body Betrayed: A Deeper Understanding of Women, Eating Disorders, and Treatment. Carlsbad, CA: Gurze Books.

Tammy Beasley, RD, CSSD, LD
Rev It Up Fitness, LLC

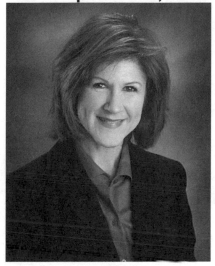

BIOGRAPHY:

Consultant, speaker, adjunct professor, Spinning instructor, and registered dietitian, Tammy Beasley brings years of qualified experience to her work. She is a certified eating disorder specialist in nutrition through the International Association of Eating Disorders Professionals since 1993, and was the first Alabama dietitian certified in sports dietetics with the American Dietetic Association in 2006. She is an active member of the Dean's Advisory Board for the College of Human Sciences, Auburn University. She is the founder and creator of Rev It Up!, which originated in 2001 and has been or is currently offered in a class format in 25 states within the U.S

Following her graduation with high honors from Auburn University and a dietetic internship with the University of Alabama in Birmingham (UAB), Tammy has been associated with some of the top health and wellness facilities in Miami, Florida, as well as Birmingham and Huntsville, Alabama. In 1995, she was selected Florida's Recognized Young Dietitian of the Year for her work with her professional associations (President of the Miami Dietetic Association) and the Miami community. After moving back home to Alabama in 1998, Tammy has served as President of the North

Alabama Dietetic Association and in various positions with the Alabama Dietetic Association, including media representative. Her work with the state culminated in her selection as Alabama's Most Outstanding Dietitian in 2007. When she is not consulting, writing, or speaking on nutrition, she can be found on the ball field with her husband cheering for their two sons, Adam and Luke!

Visit the Web site, www.revitupfitness.com, for more information on Tammy and the history of Rev It Up!